Tracey Cox is well-known f[...] relationships, including *The S[...] the USA), *Would Like to Meet* ([...] and *Date Patrol* (Discovery in[...] *Cosmopolitan* and radio show [...] *Oprah*, CNN and *The Today Show* in the USA, as well as numerous prime time UK chat shows. She has an academic background in psychology and has counselled via the media for more than fifteen years. She's sold well over a million books, six of which are also international bestsellers. Her first book, *Hot Sex*, was an instant worldwide success and is now available in 140 countries and translated into more than twenty languages. Other titles include *supersex, superdate, superflirt, Hot Relationships, The Sex Inspector's Masterclass, Quickies* and *superhotsex*. Tracey is UK *Glamour* magazine's relationships coach and has a weekly column in *Closer* magazine as well as contributing to a variety of other publications. Tracey is also resident 'sexpert' for ivillage.com and has her own range of sex toys and products.

Check out her website www.traceycox.com

What the critics say about Tracey and her books:

'The power to transform your sex life from average to outstanding overnight'
FHM

'Tracey Cox is stunningly well informed about sex. She can tell a G-spot from an A-spot and could probably find both of them before the rest of us have got the map references'
The Mirror

'What distinguishes Cox is at the heart of her appeal: the ability to talk about sex in a universal way'
The Times

'Frank, forthright and at times hysterically funny'
Cosmopolitan

THE SEX DOCTOR

FIX YOUR LOVE LIFE FAST

TRACEY COX

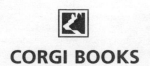

CORGI BOOKS

TRANSWORLD PUBLISHERS
61–63 Uxbridge Road, London W5 5SA
a division of The Random House Group Ltd
www.booksattransworld.co.uk

THE SEX DOCTOR
A CORGI BOOK: 9780552153409

First publication in Great Britain

Corgi edition published 2007

Addresses for Random House Group Ltd companies outside the UK
can be found at: www.randomhouse.co.uk
The Random House Group Ltd Reg. No. 954009

The Random House Group Ltd makes every effort to ensure that the
papers used in its books are made from trees that have been legally sourced
from well-managed and credibly certified forests. Our paper procurement policy
can be found at: www.randomhouse.co.uk/paper.htm

Typeset in 10.5/13.5 pt Galliard
by Falcon Oast Graphic Art Ltd

Printed and bound in Great Britain by
Cox & Wyman Ltd, Reading, Berkshire.

2 4 6 8 10 9 7 5 3 1

To my mother Shirley, who has a gloriously open and non-judgemental attitude to sex, and my sister Deborah, who shared her impressive knowledge of all things sexual, thanks to a career with Family Planning.

Both of you have been remarkably influential and helpful in my choice of career – and in my life.

With deepest gratitude – I love you both very much.

Contents

Acknowledgements   ix
Introduction   xi

1 SEX FOR SINGLES   1
Get more of it, make the most of it

2 HOW GOOD ARE YOU IN BED?   38
And how to be much, much better

3 THE NITTY-GRITTY   75
Hot new techniques to try

4 NOW *THAT* HIT THE SPOT!   107
How to orbit *your* orgasms

5 SORTING SEX DILEMMAS   142
Solutions for when your heart and other parts can't
agree

6 COUPLE'S CLIMAX CLINIC   172
Lust for the long haul

7 SAME-SEX STUFF   219
The latest on gay, lesbian and bi sex – with tons of
tips for straights as well

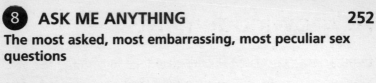

8 ASK ME ANYTHING 252
The most asked, most embarrassing, most peculiar sex questions

Useful Contacts and Resources 288
Index 292

Acknowledgements

Writing *The Sex Doctor* feels like coming home for me. Transworld are the people who published my first book, *Hot Sex: How to Do it*, launching me into a much-loved writing career. Diana Beaumont, the editor of this book, was also the editor of the first and is largely responsible for me living in the UK and for my books being published worldwide. Diana was the first person outside Australia, where *Hot Sex* was originally published, to buy the book for the UK market – and as it turned out, it was the first book she bought for the company! It seems fitting that eight years later we are still a team, not to mention bloody good friends. So an enormous thanks to you, Di, for doing such a superb job of editing this one as well!

I would also like to thank retrospectively Nerrilee Weir of Random House Australia. Nerrilee is the Rights Manager responsible for selling *Hot Sex* worldwide. It's now in 140 countries and if Nerrilee didn't manage to sell it, it's because they don't read books there. A big thank you in advance to the many Transworld and Random House people who I know will work hard to make sure this book is a success. Thanks to Karen Reid in Australia, Publicity Manager and still one of my very best friends, despite us living on different sides of the world. And to the big bosses in the UK: the effervescent Bill Scott-Kerr, Martin Higgins (who gets better looking every time I see him!) and Larry Finlay, who has always believed in me and been a true friend as well as a brilliant publisher.

Gushing thanks to everyone who shared intimate details of their sex lives for this book: Hazel Steward, Kathy Greenberg, Thamilini Nagaratnam and Fabienne Segarra (who also happens to be my highly addictive hairdresser). Thanks also to my adored *Sex Inspector* sidekick, Michael Alvear, and his gorgeous partner Robert Dajksler; and to Victoria Lehmann, sex therapist and lovely friend, for casting an experienced eye over some chapters.

Thanks from the bottom of my heart to my family, as always. I've dedicated this book to my mother and sister, but the rest of you shouldn't feel left out. You are all so supportive and precious to me – Shirley, Terry, Patrick, Maureen, Nigel, Diana, Deborah, Doug, Charlie and Maddy.

For keeping me sane, making me laugh and always being there for me, a *ginormous* thanks to my lovely friends, especially Sam Brick, Rachel Corcoran, Claire Faragher, Sandra Aldridge, Peggy Bunker and Catherine Jarvie. Anyone who's read my acknowledgements in previous books knows how important, loved and appreciated my agent and dear friend Vicki McIvor is. Vicki, thanks never, ever seems enough for all you do for me.

My humblest thanks also to my readers. Some of you write to me via my website to tell me how much you like my books and it never fails to make me puff up with pride when you say they made a difference.

Finally, huge thanks to the magazines and website who allowed me to use some small sections from previously published material. Some of the information contained in this book originally appeared in *Glamour*, *Closer* and on www.ivillage.com.

Introduction

A fantastic sex life isn't the norm, it's a rarity. Modern life makes it difficult for just about all of us. Whether we're two weeks, two months or two years into a relationship, we've got high expectations of both our sex and love lives, and the inclination and ability to walk away when things get tough. And they do get tough. For everyone.

In the beginning, we're all a bit smug and convinced the clichés aren't going to apply to us. But then they do, and you can stomp about saying 'Bugger!' all you like, but it's not going to change the situation. Reading this book, however, just might. I know that sounds a bit up myself – I'm not, truly – but I'm really quite chuffed with the information contained in *The Sex Doctor*! Like all my other books, the techniques have been road-tested by real couples and their response hasn't just been good, it's been bloody impressive – some of them didn't come out for weeks!

I learned a lot researching this book, and if *I'm* discovering new things – having read, written and talked about sex pretty much constantly for the last fifteen years – the chances are you'll learn something too. The thing is, sex and intimacy are grown-up skills and most of us, sadly, are still in junior high.

So how do you become a better lover? Advice like 'just be yourself' is silly. People used to tell me that when I was nervous about doing live TV, and I'd always think, *which* self exactly? Do I go on air as the 'Tracey who watches telly' in trackpants, toothpaste-stained T-shirt and no makeup, casually putting my feet up on the couch? Or do I go on as 'Tracey out on the town', slightly tipsy, talking too much and too loudly and probably showing too much leg? Saying 'just be yourself' in bed is just as unhelpful, besides, being yourself is sometimes the problem.

How good we are in bed is heavily dependent on the experiences we've had so far in life. If yours have left you bitter, cynical and selfish about sex, being yourself clearly isn't going to thrill the knickers off your partner! So I'm not going to tell you to do that. Instead, I'm going to give you a rundown of all the latest research and the new, outside-the-box ways of thinking about sex, packaged in a (hopefully) entertaining, practical and useful format. There's stuff for you to ponder, advice that will reassure, saucy tips and techniques you can try instantly, long-term fix-its and more than the odd lecture designed to prod you out of being lazy. Most of all, though, this book aims to make people feel good about themselves sexually. This was the prime focus of sex pioneer Alfred Kinsey, who in my opinion is still the world's most influential researcher of our time. *The Sex Doctor* seeks to continue what Kinsey started. Let's hear it for a world where sex is something we celebrate, rather than tut-tut and generally disapprove of.

Happy reading (not to mention other things)!

1 Sex for Singles

Get more of it, make the most of it

• •

Being single gets bad press, particularly if you're female. Ask people to conjure up an image of a single woman and Bridget Jones comes to mind: a plump, lonely, late-night ice-cream scoffer whose two best friends are wine and cigarettes. Men fare slightly better – at least there's the dashing, if bordering on sleazy, player hovering alongside the man in the cardigan, hair slicked and parted down the middle, nostrils and ears attractively sprouting hair. Yes, the general impression of 'single' is definitely one of barren unhappiness, punctuated by daily bouts of desperate sobbing, TV dinners for one and phones which are watched but never ring.

But there's something horribly wrong with this picture: no single person I know fits the bill. My single friends are gorgeous, gregarious, fun-loving creatures who spend their Saturday nights wickedly flirting and flitting about fabulous bars, restaurants, clubs or parties. Yes, they might have the odd moan but 90 per cent of the time they're happy, and for good reason . . .

Let's be honest here, while sex in a long-term relationship

can often be ho-hum, sex when you're single and on a roll can be bloody marvellous! By merrily playing the field, you can enjoy a potent combination of sporadic sex (having sex on tap tends to dampen desire) and new flesh (the ultimate aphrodisiac for almost all of us). The end result is a dangerously high libido. Life is fun! When relationships aren't serious, they're zero effort and maximum laughs because you don't stick around long enough to hit problems. You don't have to work hard at sex, either, because the newness factor keeps everything hot and steamy.

As a sexy singleton you've also got the opportunity to sample different sexual styles: everybody makes love differently and experience means you'll discover your true sexual personality. Sure, sex with someone you love is special and ultimately more satisfying, but no-strings sex with someone who's so delicious you have to pick your tongue up off the floor is pretty damn special too. Far from wallowing in their aloneness, plenty of singletons are revelling in one of the lustiest times of their lives.

It's your choice what category you fall into during your single days – sad or sassy – but don't let anyone tell you differently: it's not about what you look like, it's about having the right attitude. And the right attitude is to enjoy it while you can.

This chapter tackles the dilemmas a typical single person faces, everything from how to get laid more often to advice on what to do if the person you've got earmarked for long-term turns out to be the worst lover you've ever come across (or not). But don't let me interrupt your social life, read this on a Monday night when you're not out enjoying yourself.

HOW ATTRACTIVE ARE YOU?

On a scale of one to ten, how would you rate yourself? If you're typical of the general population, whatever number you assign yourself won't reflect your true worth because most of us aren't even close to objective when judging our own looks. We're capricious – one minute we think we look great, the next we don't. And surprise, surprise, women in particular see faults when they look in the mirror. One reason our perception of ourselves is flawed is because we fail to look at the big picture, whereas people looking in on us do.

How attractive we think we are influences our choice of partner: we tend to match up with people who rate the same as us. If you think you're a three, you're not going to feel comfortable lying next to a nine; a nine doesn't usually hook up with a three because they feel short-changed. The social exchange theory says people like to maximize their rewards and minimize the costs. 'Could I do better?' is a thought which plagues almost all of us at some stage in a relationship, and we don't stop asking ourselves this, even when we're married with three kids. The question is: Have *you* got the relationship *you* deserve?

Rate yourself

- **Do you worry about what you look like?** Attractive people tend to be more conscious of their appearance. But what came first, the chicken or the egg? Are they self-conscious because people look at them more often? Or attractive because they're vain and spend a lot of time on their appearance? Interestingly, people who worry about their looks tend to think they're a lot less attractive than they really are. This could be because they compare themselves with very good looking people rather than the average person.

- **How physically attractive are you?** The good news is,

> 'On a girly night, my girl-friends and I all wrote down three adjectives which best described everyone around the table. It was the biggest ego boost we'd ever had and fascinating to see what we all saw in each other but not in ourselves.'
>
> Vicki, 28

unless you've got the ego of Donald Trump, you're almost certainly better looking than you think. People don't focus on your faults half as much as you think they do because they're too busy worrying about their own. If you're female, are paranoid about your body and feel slightly uncomfortable in public, you're almost certainly hotter than you think for all the reasons listed above.

> **Want to find out what others think of you? www.hotornot.com invites people to submit anonymous photos of themselves for others to rate out of ten. It's been so popular it clocked up nearly 2 million daily page views within a week of launching.**

Another clue as to how attractive you are is to look at your partner or past partners. Subconsciously we tend to match up with people we think are similar physically, though as we get older or get to know the person better, looks become less important. If you're rich and powerful deduct points as both these qualities guarantee you'll attract people far better looking than you are.

- **What's your social standing?** The cooler your job and the more money you earn, the more attractive you are to others. Ditto if you're famous. Sadly, intelligence and academic achievement can actually work against you if you're female. Some men, but not all, thank God, are threatened by this (wimps).

- **How emotionally intelligent are you?** This will score you points with people looking for long-term partners. Being honest, loyal, caring and sensitive are all valued. Emotional intelligence is also the area we have the most control over. It's a lot easier to vow to be kind than to vow to be an Oscar winner in six months' time.

- **Are you outgoing and gregarious?** We notice people who make themselves known to us and by proxy find them more attractive. Our personality plays a huge factor in how attractive we are and big personalities usually rate higher than shy, wallflower types. Humour also plays a part. We all know the unattractive but funny guy who always lands the best-looking girl at the party. But while humorous men are seen as more attractive by women, studies show amusing women aren't necessarily more attractive to men.

- **How old are you?** This is a weird one because at a certain stage in your life youth is seen as attractive, later on age might work for you. Older men sometimes pull more attractive women because they're more accomplished. Despite being far less ageist than previous generations, most of us still look for someone within five years of our age. In the past, women would date five years older, and men five years younger but these days it doesn't tend to matter which sex has blown out more candles. Interestingly, while there's still a general perception that young women are more attractive than older, it depends totally on how good you look. Given the choice between a hot-looking older woman and a not-so-hot younger one, most men will opt for Mrs Robinson – and be pleasantly surprised. Many women gain confidence with age, know what they need sexually and aren't scared to ask for it.

  > *What do women most want? To have more energy, be a size 10 forever and look ten years younger, according to a study of 3,000 women aged twenty-five to fifty.*

- **Are you protective and supportive?** Women still look for men who can provide for them and some men are still quite keen on having a 'little woman' tucked away at home providing back-up. The exception being wealthy women – because they don't need to rely on men for money, they tend to pick their partners for the reasons lots of men do: youth and looks.

Make yourself more attractive instantly:

- **Think of yourself as more attractive:** If you think you look good, you move and behave more confidently, which means others perceive you as more attractive.
- **Hang around ugly people:** It's called the contrast effect. We feel pretty around ugly people and ugly around pretty people. The good news is you don't have to switch friends if they're attractive because it also works the other way around . . .

- **Hang around pretty people:** This works in a different way. We're defined by our friends and peer group and the cooler and better-looking they are, the cooler and better-looking we appear to others. This is assuming, of course, that you have a healthy self-esteem that lets you realize you're as good as the others.

- **Don't idealize:** Women in particular, compare themselves to an ideal standard of beauty (genetic freaks called supermodels). If asked to rate something like our interpersonal skills, however, we measure ourselves against the norm rather than compare ourselves with Freud. In one study, researchers got men and women to sit a simple mathematical exam. Both sexes scored evenly. Then they repeated the exercise, but got everyone to do it in their bathing suits. Forced to sit there in a bikini, the women's results dived while the men's didn't alter. Instead of concentrating

> **!** *If you're on the curvy side and want to be seen as slimmer, linger over pre-dinner activities rather than the traditional coffee at your place afterwards. It seems hunger affects men's preferences for body type. Asked to rate photos of women in leotards with faces blanked out, students on their way to dinner rated the larger women more attractive than those students who'd just eaten.*

on the problem in hand, women concentrated on other women's bodies, checking out how they measured up, as well as wondering how the men were rating them.

- **Show people you like them:** We like people who like us. The easiest way to make yourself more appealing to others is to be friendly and warm.
- **Get older:** There's evidence that people feel more attractive with age, even if they don't look it.

SOLUTIONS TO THINGS LOTS OF SINGLES STRUGGLE WITH

Sex and snog buddies: A good idea?

Most of us have either had one or have one: the old faithful who can always be counted on if all else fails for either a good snog and snuggle or damn good (and usually very wicked) sex. So why we don't actually date these people? Sometimes it's because one of you is already involved with someone else (naughty), while other times it's a grown-up realization that as much as you're fond of each other, you don't have enough in common outside the bedroom to make it work.

If you've got the right personality for it and are both single, I think sex and snog buddies (SB's) can be a very good idea. Having someone you can cuddle when you're drunk/down/just feel like it, quells 'skin hunger': the simple need to be touched and held by another person. The snog part reminds us how good kissing and sexual affection are and helps us feel sexy and attractive. Having a snog buddy means the 'drought' between partners leaves us a lot less parched and panicky than we would be without someone's lips attached to ours on the odd occasion. Sex buddies serve an extra purpose: they provide a safe, sexual outlet and stop us taking risks with someone we shouldn't. If you're a horny little thing and are tempted to hump your workmate's legs when deprived of a bit, sex buddies are a very good idea indeed. Much better to sleep with someone you know than head down to your local with £20 in your pocket and a nasty gleam in your eye. We tend to use condoms with SBs or both get tested and use condoms with other people, until the point when either of you meets someone you want to be faithful to. And no, you can't keep them when this happens. The point of having an SB is null and void once you have sex on tap, and continuing it means you're no longer SBs, you're having an affair. There's a huge difference between an affair and a rather agreeable arrangement for consequence-free, high-quality sex with someone you're quite attached to.

Like all good things, however, there is a downside to the SB thing. As much as the *Sex and the City* girls rate them – 'They're a shot in the arm for sexual self-esteem,' Carrie enthuses – there's a temptation for one of you to make more of the relationship at some point, which is when you could find out that it's possible to find someone stimulating in bed but boring out of it. Either that or you end up falling for them and the feeling isn't reciprocated, or vice versa. Either way, it means the sex is ruined for ever. Don't do it.

Is it wrong to sleep with someone on the first night if you want more than a one-night stand?

It's not wrong but it's risky. If you want to up your chances of the relationship being healthy and lasting the distance, do the opposite: try to put off having full, penetrative sex for as long as possible. Not because 'good girls don't' or because he might judge you, even though he may, but because you're creating the best possible circumstances for the two of you to bond physically and emotionally. Once you sleep with someone, you keep on sleeping with them. Which means you're instantly, and literally, intimately bonded, which effectively robs you of logic and objectivity. 'Lust blindness' causes us to get so involved with our partner's body, we forget to look closely at the person inside. This is what's usually happened when someone pleads 'But I love him!', when 'love' has landed them in hospital. No-one deliberately sets out to fall in love with a bastard, you end up there because you rushed into something too fast and didn't do your homework. Sex is a strong glue and it holds together the most unlikely of couples. The longer you avoid doing it, the more time you'll spend out of the bedroom, talking and finding out if that person is right for you. Besides, waiting teaches you both the merits of sexual anticipation, and taking baby steps – kissing first, then touching, then oral sex – teaches you that sex doesn't have to mean intercourse. In the *Story of O*, the main character was taught only to let a man make love to one bit of her body at a time, so he'd truly learn how to pleasure each and every part of her.

What if I only want a one-night stand?

You little player, you! Only joking, it's fine to just want sex, so long as the person you're having it with agrees. Call me old-fashioned, idealistically hopeful or plain deluded, but as much as I don't expect you to stand at the foot of someone's bed and announce solemnly, 'I'm just here for the sex', I don't think it's too much to ask for you to send out strong signals saying pretty much that. And that means no whispering sweet nothings unless they're sexual, no saying how fabulous they are, unless you're talking about physical attributes, no hinting at future plans – 'I'll have to take you there someday'. In other words, make all your chat-up sexual rather than romantic. This sends a clear, unsullied message. If you're really nice, you'll say something like, 'Look, you turn me on something dreadful but I can't really promise anything. Do you want to/can I stay the night or would that be out of order?'. This spells out your intentions in a light-hearted way, and if they agree, your conscience is pretty clear.

THE TOP FIVE THINGS HE'S HOPING YOU'LL DO THE FIRST TIME YOU HAVE SEX

- **Give great oral sex:** it's not only one of his favourite things, it shows you're as interested in giving as you are in receiving pleasure.

- **Be active:** I'm not suggesting you bounce around the bed like a four-year-old who's just consumed their body weight in sweets, but please don't leave it up to him to make all the moves.

- **Not stress about your body:** Hiding under the covers, insisting the lights are turned out – you know the drill. Even if your thighs look like orange peel, you're having sex with the man, and unless it's a one-night stand, at some point he's going to have to see you naked. Get it over with and done with: let him see everything first time around and you'll both feel better.

- **Let him know you're enjoying it:** Listen, he's read the girls' mags and maybe even picked up the odd sex book or two. He knows women fake it and it's not that easy to get everything right. Don't patronize him by pretending you like everything he does (unless of course you do – lucky cow!) but do let him know when he's doing something particularly well. A moan or '*ummmm*' will do.

- **Save the post-sex emotional fallout for your girlfriends:** If he really doesn't want to know you now that he's had his wicked way, you'll only embarrass yourself by trying to find out if you're an item. If he really likes you, he'll call the next day and organize your next date. The more relaxed you are about the whole thing, the more smitten he'll be. Be affectionate and shoot a few meaningful looks, so he knows it meant something, but resist hanging onto his legs as he makes for the front door.

How important is it to feel chemistry for your partner?

If you want a passionate, intense relationship, it's crucial. If the word 'content' makes you feel warm and fuzzy rather than ancient and anxious, not so. Chemistry changes the dynamics of a relationship, making it more intense and therefore more dangerous, which isn't everyone's idea of fabulous. It's perfectly possible to click with someone and have a lovely time together without ever feeling 'chemistry' with that person, and controlled, sensible relationships suit some people. If, however, you're after a more powerful emotional and sexual experience, by all means go for the person you want to slam up against a wall and swap souls and saliva with. Chemistry won't guarantee you lifetime love, but it's a bloody good start, and it's likely to make you stick around for the finish. Even good relationships have massive boring bits and chemistry is what keeps us there, picking our fingernails and waiting to see if things improve, rather than dashing out the door the second problems start.

What if I'm enjoying being single and playing the field so much I don't want to settle down?

This is a bit like asking how long is a piece of string. If you're twenty-one-years old with no dependants this clearly isn't a problem. If you're forty years old, female and want children, it may be. If you're thirty-five and about to lose the love of your life because you can't commit past next Saturday night, it definitely is. In other words, it depends very much on your age, circumstances and the reasons why you want to stay single.

You're young, freshly dumped and hurting, have just come out of a long-term relationship which went horribly wrong, having too much fun, not sure what sort of person will suit you long-term: these are all healthy reasons for

THE TOP FIVE THINGS SHE'S HOPING YOU'LL DO THE FIRST TIME YOU HAVE SEX

- **Give great oral sex:** Given that it's how most women orgasm, showing you like doing it and, even better, know how to do it well, scores big points. It also shows you're not squeamish about sex.

- **Compliment her:** Even if it's a mumbled 'Perfect breasts!' or 'God, your skin feels amazing', make some acknowledgement of the fact that you're thrilled to have finally got your hands on her gorgeous bod.

- **Focus on foreplay:** Spend lots of time kissing, pay attention to her breasts, tease her, feel her through her panties. If you dive straight for the good bits, or worse try to penetrate after just a few minutes, you'll be lucky if you have sex at all.

- **Have an orgasm:** Yes, there are many reasons why it sometimes has nothing to do with her (see pages 206–10), but in her slightly altered condition (forget the alcohol, it's vulnerability which is doing it) she'll interpret it as you not finding her attractive or not being good in bed. So if you don't orgasm and you're comfortable talking about it, say something afterwards like 'Look, don't think you don't turn me on. The reason I didn't orgasm was because . . .' (I had too much to drink/your cat was staring at me).

- **Say something nice afterwards:** If you really, really like her, say something like 'That was exactly what I'd hoped it would be. I think you're amazing'. If you're keen but not that keen, at least let her know you want to see her again and make a date before you leave. Even if it's a one-night stand and you want to just get out of there, do the decent thing. Say 'I really enjoyed wanting to stay single for a bit (or lot) longer. So is wanting to be single permanently, if that's what you honestly prefer. The whole marriage-and-kids-thing isn't for everyone and there's nothing wrong with you if you don't want to chase that dream. I know people who have decided long-term relationships simply aren't for them. They don't like having to answer to people and don't consider the intimacy of monogamy to be a fair trade for what they see as the inevitable boredom of a relationship.

When wanting to stay single *can* be a problem is if you're hurting yourself or others. Consider whether you're really enjoying being single or if it's a way of keeping people at arm's length because you've got intimacy issues. Has the term 'commitment phobe' been flung at you rather a lot, perhaps along with the drink the person was holding? In short, are you staying single from a position of strength or is it fear that keeps you that way because you're terrified of letting people get close to you in case you get hurt. If this is making you feel a little uncomfortable, it's probably true. If you want to do something about it, I'd recommend taking a long look at your childhood for clues as to why commitment

Most people in the US are waiting until they're older to get married. US Census data shows the median age of a woman's first marriage has increased six years from 20 to 26 since 1970. A commonly cited reason for the delay is that they're waiting to find a soulmate.

seems like a bad idea to you. What happened to you, or what did you see that's subconsciously made you think falling in love and staying with someone isn't safe? Ask old friends or siblings for some insight. Perhaps it isn't linked to your childhood but to something that happened as an adult. A broken heart is pretty effective at making us shy away from future commitment, and so is discovering that a much-loved partner had an affair. Identifying the problem is a big step towards solving it. If you feel you need further help, read up on the topic (the bookstores are heaving with stuff on this) or consider seeing a good counsellor for a few sessions.

F FOR HER

Five good reasons to stop panicking about finding 'Mr Right'

- It's likely that some of the best, most wicked sex you'll have is with someone you don't love. Most women don't do the really kinky stuff with a man they think could be a future husband.
- The longer you leave it, the fussier you'll be – this is a good thing because it means you're not 'settling'.
- The longer you stay single, the more independent you'll be. This means you'll choose a life partner for the right reasons: you *want* them rather than *need* them.
- The more Mr Wrongs you go out with, the more likely you are to find Mr Right. The more you veer away from type, the more likely you are to find someone who'll make you happy.
- For every successful single woman who regrets having focused on her career, there's a woman who settled down too early and thinks she's missed out. There's an up and down side to everything.

HELP! I'M A MIDDLE-AGED MALE VIRGIN!
Why and what to do if it's you

He was twenty-eight and gorgeous. I was thirty-two, newly single, nicely inebriated and eager to get the dinner over with to find out if the deliciously sexy kisses we'd been having were a hint of things to come. 'I read a story today about how people are finally taking AIDS seriously and getting regular tests,' I said (as good a way as any to let him know the whole condom thing wasn't negotiable). Jason looked down and toyed with his food, saying nothing. 'Have you been tested?' I prompted. 'No,' he answered, 'I don't need to be'. Ah, a devout condom-user. 'So, you've never slept with anyone without a condom?' I countered, ready to launch into my it-only-takes-one spiel. 'Well, no. I haven't even used a condom. I'm a virgin.' Huh? I paused, fork in mid-air, and looked at him. No, he couldn't be, not looking like that. Then he blushed. Ohmigod, he bloody well is! What the hell was I supposed to do now?

Innocent, untouched, eager to please – for some women, taking a man's virginity is the ultimate erotic experience. I just felt a heavy, suffocating cloak of responsibility settle on my shoulders. I'd just come out of a marriage and didn't want a long-term relationship. But I *did* want sex – and how many dates would we have to go on before he felt comfortable enough to 'do it'? Did he expect me to marry him afterwards? Wasn't that what virgins expected?

'Why?' I asked him.

'I decided to save myself for someone special,' he said. *Please God let me not be her.* 'And I think I'm looking at her right now.' He beamed. *Oh great.* I gave a watery smile and we limped along for a few more dates, but I ended up confessing that I didn't want to be 'The One'. 'You deserve better,' I said a trifle dramatically, 'someone who will appreciate you having waited all this time'.

'I agree,' he said.

Oh. Moving right along then . . .

The moral of that little tale, guys, is that this is what you're going to be up against – or not, as the case may be (sorry, couldn't resist). Women are going to make several assumptions when/if they find out you're a virgin: a) that they can't just have their wicked way with you and exit stage left (even though that's probably your idea of heaven, b) that there's something wrong with you (your worst fear), c) that you're probably not going to be the best lay she's ever had (this, I'm afraid, is probably true since practice does make perfect). I'm not trying to upset you by telling you this, I'm being super-honest so you don't get any nasty surprises. If I demystify the whole thing, you can tackle it (and her).

> 'I think most women have slept with virgins – you just don't know it because most of us don't own up to it. Remember that guy you thought was a little inexperienced? It was probably his first time.'
>
> John, 19

How did it happen?

Some of you have deliberately remained a virgin. Perhaps you're religious and don't believe in sex before marriage. Maybe you're like Jason and see sex as something special and don't want to dilute it with several partners. Maybe you want to marry a virgin and figure if you expect her to be, you should be too. In most cases though, it's not deliberate: you just missed the point when everyone else did 'it'. Maybe your girlfriend was less keen on putting out than other girls. Maybe you were less sure of what to do than other guys, so you didn't push it. Maybe you were shy or didn't find it that easy to get a girlfriend until much later than everyone else. Then you were still a virgin and none of your friends were, so you felt a little hung up about it. It becomes a big deal, you're terrified you'll embarrass yourself, so avoid making any sexual advances at all. Girls aren't used to men *not* wanting to sleep with them so you quickly get a reputation of being 'a bit weird' or 'gay', and before you know it you're scared even of dating. You can't talk to your friends about it because you figure it's such a hideous secret and relationships seem like they'd be too stressful to bother with because if it was bad being an eighteen-year-old virgin, being a twenty-eight-year-old one is even worse . . . and before you know it, you've ended up where you are now. Reaching middle-age as a virgin.

Why does everyone think all male virgins are ugly, nerdy or shy?

Because society tends to view men as sex-crazed – willing, able and ready to have sex with anything that stands still for longer than a minute. If you haven't done it by the age of twenty-five, thirty or forty people *will* think you're odd. And because it's unusual to be a virgin over the age of twenty-one, gossip travels fast. I guarantee that if you tell even one person in your circle of friends, they will *all* know within two days – it's way too juicy to keep to themselves. 'It's become such a joke among my friends that when I do start talking to a woman, they give me a really hard time and I never get anywhere,' says Craig, one male virgin I spoke to. 'They make me feel like I'm not part of the club. I used to think women might find it a turn-on to want to teach a virgin, but it's not true, I'm considered a freak. Women are either shocked or they laugh. I don't try to hide it because I'm well aware it'll become painfully obvious once we hit the bedroom.'

Some older male virgins *are* a bit nerdy. If you feel inept, don't know how to flirt and don't feel you can go to a party and interact successfully with women or men, it's hard to get yourself in a position where you get the opportunity to lose your virginity. You need to be socially skilled to get a date these days.

Don't some women get turned on by it?

Yes, the news isn't all bad! Some women will find you being a virgin a huge turn on. Jennifer, an attractive twenty-eight-year-old lawyer I know, seduced a friend's son two years ago and claims it was 'the most erotic, mind-blowing' thing she's ever done, though possibly not the most moral. 'I've deliberately gone out with young guys since then hoping to strike it lucky,' she says, 'unfortunately, though, male virgins over fifteen aren't too thick on the ground.'

Another friend is the only woman her husband has ever slept with, even though she's bedded over twenty men. 'He's five years younger than me and totally devoted,' she says. 'I didn't trust other guys, but this time I know he won't play around. When you're the first woman he's slept with, he's emotionally yours for life.' These women, and others, claim being the first to introduce a man to the pleasures of sex is the ultimate in sexual head-games, a lusty sensation unlike anything else they've experienced.

'It's a turn-on both physically and emotionally. I think it's the power you have,' says Jennifer. 'The rush I get from knowing he's never seen a woman naked before, never touched a woman's breast or been inside her. Sometimes I'll orgasm even before he does!'

> 'I was incredibly turned on by the prospect of taking his virginity but I don't think he was. He was very nervous but once we got over that first time he turned out to be an excellent lover. He got right into it and was really innovative.'
>
> Jane, 26

Power isn't the only appeal. Being able to play teacher and not be judged on your sexual expertise are also pluses of sleeping with a male virgin. Virgins pay attention and listen. There are a lot of guys out there who think they're great lovers when they're not. When you try to guide them or tell them they're doing something wrong, they get offended. With a virgin, it's usually different.

You look to your partner to teach you, and with time and patience she can mould you into her idea of the perfect lover.

So how do I lose it?

There is an argument for just getting it out of the way any way you can. This might mean having a one-night stand with someone you wouldn't necessarily want to date (remembering to always wear a condom of course) or it might mean paying for it (see 'Paying for Sex', pages 20–1). I know several men who have done either of these things and I'd probably do the same if I was in that situation. However, it may not suit you. After all this time, you might figure it's worth waiting until you meet someone you really like, or perhaps you've already met her and are reading this in a blind panic, desperate to know what to do. Well it just so happens that you're in luck, because that's exactly what I'm about to tell you.

First up, the obvious question: do you tell her or not? If you do, you risk her feeling freaked out and possibly running away. If you don't, you might embarrass yourself by being the worst lover she's ever had or ejaculating before you even get to do the deed. There's no hard and fast rule for this (even if you might be); the best advice I can give is that it depends on the relationship. If she's warm and loving, I'd tell her. If she's quite sassy and you're a little in awe of her and not sure of her reaction, don't. If it's all over and done with in the first thrust, just blame it on her being so damn gorgeous.

Inexperience doesn't necessarily mean less pleasure for her – it can be the opposite. As a virgin, you'll probably try harder. Let's face it, you don't have to be a rocket scientist to be great in bed. Educate yourself by reading a few decent sex books, let her guide you if you've confessed and you'll figure it out pretty quickly. An effective way to get around the problem of ejaculating too soon is to masturbate just before you see her that evening, à la *There's Something About Mary*, so you'll be less sensitive. If you're really worried, masturbate twice: once in the afternoon and once just before you walk out the door to meet her. Tell her it's unlikely you'll last long (you're a virgin/so turned on by her – depending on what your story is) but there's always a second time, and a third, and a fourth.

PAYING FOR SEX: WHY SOMETIMES IT'S A GOOD IDEA

Sex workers provide a very necessary service, and be warned, this little box of information isn't going to be terribly PC. I believe, for instance, that if someone is going to be unfaithful to their partner, it's sometimes more forgivable if they've done it with a sex worker than someone they might be likely to forge a relationship with.

Why would they need to? Sometimes people desperately want to try something a little 'out there' sexually, but don't want to do it with their partner. They respect them too much or don't want their partner to know. Sometimes, it's is a one-off wish: after they've done it, the appeal disappears or they can use that one experience as fantasy fodder from there on. If the sex worker is understanding, a condom is used and all precautions taken, it can offer a solution to a potentially big problem which might otherwise split the couple up. I'm not saying I'd be particularly happy if my partner did this, it's just something to consider.

Another time I would heartily condone someone visiting a sex worker is to lose their virginity if they're starting to stress about it (see 'Middle-aged male virgins' on pages 15–20). In some parts of Europe, it used to be customary for a father to send his son to a madam at the age of sixteen and she would deflower him and teach him how to make love to a woman properly. There's a lot to be said for that custom – not only did the son get a practical lesson in how to be a great lover, he was able to lose his virginity in a safe environment, away from ridicule.

Another instance where I think it's acceptable is for people who are bordering on elderly with partners who are chronically ill. If your partner can't and never will be able to have sex again, it doesn't mean your needs and desires disappear. Often an understanding person will give permission for them to seek sex elsewhere, and it's a lot easier emotionally knowing they are having sex for sex's sake, rather than seeing someone on the side and falling for them.

A few words of caution, if you intend to visit a sex worker, it's best if you stick to larger, reputable organizations rather than pick up someone off the street. A lot of brothels are slickly run businesses: check out advertisements for them and choose the biggest one. They're probably making the most money and have the most to lose if their clients aren't satisfied. In big, successful brothels, the girls are kept safe and tested regularly for STI's. *Obviously* you should still use a condom (read the 'Things you don't want to know but must' section on pages 34-6) and be extremely careful about being seen entering or leaving the premises. Don't use your credit card, pay cash, and if you don't want anyone to find out, don't tell anyone. And I mean *anyone*. This is your business, no-one else's.

I would write something about women paying for sex and argue its merits, except that, even with the efforts of the experienced and industrious Heidi Fleiss, brothels-for-women just don't take off. Maybe it's easier for us to get sex without having to pay, maybe we don't like the concept of it or maybe we're just tight. (And not in a good way!) Either way, despite all the Calvin Klein underwear types lounging around for women to choose from, they seem oddly unappealing when they come with a price tag. Put the same men in a cool bar after midnight and it's another story – and it's not just the money. Honest!

One common mistake you need to be wary of is not to be too penis-centric. Because you've never done 'it', intercourse, unsurprisingly, tends to become the main focus of sex for you. Don't let it be and make sure you give her lots of foreplay. Will the earth move when you finally do get to do it? For many, no. 'I felt horribly embarrassed at my inexperience and just wanted to get it over and done with,' is the common response of many male virgins. Some say that while they certainly remember the first girl they slept with, they'd rather forget her because they associate her with feeling inadequate. On a brighter note, a lot of men say they woke the next day with a spring in their step and a weight off their shoulders. Others, who had sex with someone who really meant something to them, say it was incredibly special. As I hope your experience will be.

SHOULD YOU DUMP SOMEONE IF THEY'RE BAD IN BED?

The politically correct answer, of course, is no, but my advice would be yes – at least in some situations. The thing is, if sex isn't working at the start, you haven't got a hope long term. The chance of you turning into randy eighty-year-olds, sneaking out for a quickie behind the gardening sheds at the back of the old people's home, is about as high as me winning the next lottery draw. And I haven't bought a ticket.

If sex is hugely important to you, I really wouldn't advise you settling down with someone who'd rather watch telly or doesn't even care if they're bad in bed. The more you love sex, the stronger the argument for moving on. Having said that, if you really, really like the person, there are times when it's worth sticking around.

Can bad sex be turned into good sex? Some people decide to stay with their partner regardless, so strong are their feelings for them. If you're not quite as altruistic, the main questions you need to ask yourself are these: do they want to be better and do they care that I'm not happy? If the answer is yes to both, as a general rule the problem is solvable. Here is some advice for more specific problems:

- **High versus low libidos:** Eat, drink, sleep, sex: removing regular sex from your daily routine is as unthinkable to you as deciding not to clean your teeth any more, but you have a horrible, sneaking suspicion your partner wouldn't even notice. And if they're not frothing at the mouth for sex in the beginning, what on earth are they going to be like later? This, my friend, is called 'mismatched libidos': one wants sex more than the other. It's one of the most common sex problems experienced by couples, and while it's fixable, by God you're in for a battle. First you need to ask yourself how much you like the person? If you really like them, don't dump them, but if you're lukewarm about the whole thing, save yourself a lifetime of trying to balance sexual scales and get out now. (Planning on staying? Turn to pages 212–8 for tips to get you through.)

- **Adventurous versus conservative:** Their idea of a wild session is sexy lingerie, your version would include a lap dancer wearing it and doing a private dance for both of you. Some psychologists believe our sexual attitudes and beliefs are formed by the time we reach eighteen. That means that if you're audacious and they're not, there's not a whole lot you can do to meet in the middle. I disagree. If your partner is simply shy or inexperienced, they may not have had the opportunity to explore anything outside the norm. With a bit of encouragement, a timid lover can quickly turn into a terrific one. What's crucial is their central attitude to sex. Have they just led a sheltered life or do they secretly think sex is 'dirty' and something to be endured rather than enjoyed? If it's the former, stick around. If it's the latter, you've got to challenge their childhood and/or religious presuppositions first. This isn't an easy job. Do they want to change? Are you willing to put the work in? It's doable, but it's going to take effort.

- **Selfish versus inexperienced:** To say the sex isn't satisfying you is like saying Paris Hilton likes attention: it's a whopping understatement. Whether it's a distinct lack of foreplay or what appears to be general disinterest in your pleasure, a disengaged lover isn't great. What you need to establish here is whether your partner doesn't care a hoot whether you're fulfilled, or whether it's inexperience disguising itself as indifference. Technique can be taught. Selfish people don't want to and usually won't change. It's easy to find out which camp your partner falls into: ask them to do something for you in bed – 'Honey, I'd love it if you'd play with my breasts/give me oral for longer'. Do they respond eagerly, asking you for more feedback on everything they do? Or do they sigh, sulk or ignore your request? If it's the first, hang in there, providing you're happy to play teacher for a bit. If it's the second, put your clothes back on this instant, head for the door and don't look back. See also page 144.

> 'I'd been lusting after this girl in the office for about a year and we finally ended up getting smashed at an office party and spent a weekend together. She went from being my perfect woman to the woman I least desired. She kissed badly, treated my penis like it was something disgusting and clearly didn't like sex.'
>
> James, 42

I've just had sex with my new boyfriend and he didn't orgasm. Should I be insulted that he didn't come?

Should he be insulted that you didn't either? I'm not

psychic, it's just that very, very few women have an orgasm via intercourse the first time they have sex with a new partner – lots don't have an orgasm the other 10,000 times either, but that's another story. I know, I know, it's *much* easier for him to climax than you so it's different, but the reason behind him not coming is the same reason you didn't: the pressure is on and you're both out to impress. Penises don't like pressure. They respond by either refusing to come out to play at all (his worst nightmare), playing for approximately one minute (his second worst) or refusing to stop (yours). Not being able to climax at all is often the result of him trying desperately to avoid premature ejaculation.

If you find yourself putting down your partner in public, chances are it's in front of someone good-looking. Research shows we're far more likely to downplay their good points when talking about them to attractive, new acquaintances. We're subconsciously trying to make them seem less worth stealing.

The other common reason is drinking. A friend once asked me, perplexed, 'How do people who don't drink have sex? I'd never make that first move unless I was drunk'. Alcohol may relax inhibitions, but it also desensitizes us, deadening our feelings and relaxing our muscles, including the pubococcygeus, which is the muscle you squeeze if you want to stop peeing. That's the same muscle that you've been squeezing rhythmically, diligently doing your Kegel exercises (Kegels make your vagina tighter), so that when the moment arrives, he feels snug as a bug in a rug. Sadly, twenty-five gin and tonics will make his penis feel like the only person to turn up to a concert at the Royal Albert Hall. Don't get paranoid, though, just have sex first thing in the morning, squeeze hard and he'll be suitably impressed. Add to the equation that some men *always* take ages to orgasm – always have, always will and wouldn't even get a move on during a supermodel sex sandwich – and you'll start to see why you shouldn't be insulted. Listen, I know why your ego is dented – he's supposed to be so over- come with lust at finally being allowed to go there that it's a compliment if he finishes prematurely but it doesn't neces- sarily mean he was disappointed. Honest.

🕞 FOR HER

WHY DOESN'T ANYONE WANT TO SLEEP WITH ME?

You're decent looking, easy to get on with and chat comfort- ably to men, so how come the rest of the world seems to have a boyfriend and be enjoying lots of regular, yummy sex while you're tucking yourself in each night?

- **It's been too long between boyfriends:** If you keep on doing what you've already done, you'll get what you've already got. If you've been single for ages, without so much as a drunken, stolen snog, you need to shock your system into change. Breaking the drought not only makes you relax and think maybe you will get another boyfriend after all, it prepares you for change.

  It's not my place to tell you to get out there, grab the first half-decent guy who looks your way, flirt your bottom off and slam him against the nearest wall for a bout of tonsil-tennis and maybe a quick feel, but that could be exactly what you need. Your body and brain have forgotten what touching, kissing and sex feel like, so it's not making you get out there and find it. Try lowering your standards and consider having a few flings for the hell of it. They don't have to turn into the love of your life, they're just someone to have fun with right now. You'll send off far more relaxed, sexy vibes because you'll feel attractive and desirable again.

- **You're not sending out sexy vibes:** I went a whole six months without sex – I know, shocking – because I got so swept up in work I didn't have time for a boyfriend. After a while, I got used to not having sex and stopped thinking about it. Without making a conscious decision not to, I stopped darting cheeky glances at every good-looking guy I saw, stopped wondering if the guy reading alone in the bookstore was single, stopped masturbating: in short, I stopped being a sexual being. Before that I got asked out loads. During that period no-one came near me, although I looked exactly the same. Was it because I wasn't looking and picking up signals? Probably. Was it because I wasn't sending out any of my own? Definitely. The main reason why was this: I went off sex. If you like sex, sexiness oozes from every pore, every movement. Women who feel like sex walk with a swagger, stand with their breasts and bottoms out, with a nice curve in their backs, and cross their legs slowly and deliberately until they know every man in the place is watching. They play with their hair, dip their chins and look up through their lashes with a saucy smile – and that's just when they're paying the electricity bill.

The better you get on with your mother, the more likely you are to use condoms correctly as a teen. A survey of 1,400 teenagers showed that many put them on too late or removed them too soon, but this was far less likely if they had a close relationship with their mother.

Women who love sex smell, and not in a bad way. If you're in a state of arousal, your body is pumping out come-and-get-me hormones to any man who's not working a shift at McDonalds, and men pick it up. They're not even sure *why* they're looking at you: your pheromones are speaking to their pheromones and Mother Nature is doing her damnedest to get you to do what you were put on earth for: populate. If you're not getting sex from someone else, go solo. Masturbate every day, read sexy books, watch sexy movies, dress sexily. Focus on it, daydream about your best encounters, come up with some lurid fantasies, then get back out there.

- **You desperately need a makeover:** Too-tight clothes, try-too-hard outfits like knicker-skimming skirts and tops cut to the navel, frumpy clothes, an unflattering hairdo, clothes that highlight your bad bits and disguise your best ones: beauty might be only skin deep but packaging is incredibly important. Yes we all know it shouldn't be about what you look like, but he's never going to discover how fabulous you are unless he's attracted enough to talk to you in the first place.

There are two classic mistakes long-term singles make: paying too much attention to their appearance or not enough. Turning up to a barbecue in heels, a too dressy outfit with matching accessories and perfectly applied make-up won't have the cute single guy wanting to wrestle you on the grass. It reeks of desperation. Perfect the look of Ms Desperate when out on the town by spending the whole time looking longingly into the crowd rather than having a good old gossip with the people you're with.

Classic mistake No 2: giving up. You're the one at the glitzy cocktail party in your work suit and no make-up. After all, what's the point? No-one's going to chat you up anyway – and they won't if that's your attitude. The trick to looking sexy, attractive and approachable is to think casual sexy. If you've got the right bod, a cool pair of jeans, high heels and a sexy little top or vest will take you almost anywhere. Most big department stores have a personal shopping service, so use it and try on everything they bring you – you might be surprised at what looks fab on you. Next stop, a decent hairdresser – opt for a casual rather than overly done style – and a visit to a professional make-up place. Get them to teach you a versatile day and evening look.

Now that your look's right, examine your body language. Stand and walk straight and tall, arms loosely by your side rather than crossed. Don't hold your drink up as a barrier, hold it at waist height. Make eye contact and smile. Don't stand or sit rigidly, change position

> *Think more money will make you happier? Think again. Research says a committed relationship is what will make you most happy. The only thing better is a committed relationship with lots of sex.*

every few minutes and try not to sit or stand symmetrically. Put your weight on one leg, put your hand on your hip and tilt your head to the side. Practice sexy ways to stand, walk and sit in front of the mirror. Would you want to approach you?

- **You don't really like men:** Who me? I love men! I can hear you exclaiming from here. Why, lots of your best friends are men and you adore your brother. True. But these are men you know and trust. All it takes is a few bad experiences – a lover in your past who treated you badly, the guy you thought was really going to come through but didn't call, or simply a series of disappointing, lacklustre relationships with men who didn't make you feel fabulous – and before you know it, your core trust in men falters. You stop expecting the best and start expecting the worst, which soon becomes a self-fulfilling prophecy because your hackles are always raised. You think you're radiating cool confidence, but really you're sending out toxic waves of suspicion and aggression, designed to protect you against further hurt.

The thing is, all men aren't bastards, just as all women aren't bitches. Some men, and some women, are but here's the thing: you can control how people treat you. If you behave like a doormat, men will walk all over you. If you treat them as the enemy, they will behave like one. If, instead, you approach every guy with an open mind and assume he's a nice guy *until* proven wrong, you'll bring out the best in him. Save the I-don't-put-up-with-that speech for when he does something you won't put up with, then say your piece in a calm, no-nonsense voice without histrionics. That's what will stop men treating you badly: being calmly in control. Secure women don't attract bad boys: put yourself back in the power position and suddenly you'll have nothing to fear. Realize this, go back to liking men and they'll like you. Simple as that.

Ⓜ FOR HIM

I'm an ordinary-looking bloke – I'm not handsome but I'm not weird either – so why can't I persuade anyone to have sex with me?

Here's the deal: go out searching for sex, which is effectively what you're doing, and you will indeed find yourself home alone. The extraordinarily handsome or an ostentatious wallet-waver might score despite obviously wanting nothing other than no-strings sex, but average Joes, as you describe yourself, will almost always be rebuffed. Why? For a start, your trading power isn't high – some women consider one-off sex with someone Beckhamesque a fair trade, while others will swap for posh nosh and a limo. The majority of us tend to say no because the offer is insulting, but *not*, I suspect, for the reasons you think. Knowing someone is desperate to make love to you is nearly always a gloriously delicious, if sometimes inappropriate, compliment. What's off-putting is the anyone-would-do thing which can seep through. Having to 'persuade anyone' to sleep with you sounds wretchedly desperate and fails to honour a basic female need to feel special.

It also shows zero understanding of the female sexual psyche, dragging us back to those dark and dubious days when women 'gave' sex and men 'got' it. As we can see from the rapidly rising rate of married women indulging in just-for-sex affairs, the old way of thinking – men loved sex, women didn't – is clearly wrong. The truth is, these days, if you've approached it the right way, there should be little need for persuasion. Women now have both societal permission and opportunity to indulge in all types of sex, casual or otherwise, and she's just as likely to be gliding her hand suggestively up your inner thigh as you are hers. Getting to the point where she'll want to do this however, requires great sensitivity and skill.

The gist of it is this: women have two sides and both need seducing. Think of it as a juggling act. On one hand you've got her cerebral, virtuous side – old habits die hard – the side which needs to feel respected, admired and convinced you want *her*, not just someone sprouting breasts. Even if it is just casual sex you're negotiating, it doesn't mean it can't be honourable or done with genuine affection. On the other hand, you have the

> 'I don't know what was happening, but for eighteen months, not one girl came near me. I'd gone beyond being depressed to just accepting that no-one would ever go out with me again. Then all of a sudden, it lifted. I have no idea what caused it or what made it go away.'
>
> Charlie, 34

antithesis, the incorrigibly wicked part of her which *wants* to catch you lustfully gazing at her breasts when you think she's studying the menu. How the scales balance depends on the individual, so I can't help you there, but place too much emphasis on the wicked and she'll view you with suspicion, overplay the other and you'll be plonked in the 'friend' basket quicker than she can say 'nice guy'.

F FOR HER

CONTRACEPTION CRISIS: EMERGENCY SOLUTIONS

- **You forgot to take your pill:** Each Pill is different, so read the instructions which come with yours, though the following is good general advice. If it's an 'active' pill – not one of the white sugar pills you take during your period on a twenty-eight-day pill to keep you in the habit of taking it – it's OK to take it as soon as you remember and continue as normal as long as it's less than *twelve hours* late. If it's more than twelve hours late or you've missed more than one pill, use condoms for the next seven days. If you're at the end of your cycle and there aren't that many active pills left, skip taking the placebo period pills and start a new pack, then keep taking them through to the end of the month. If you're confused, check with a pharmacist.

- **You didn't realize you'd missed one or two pills and have already had sex:** It's one thing suddenly realizing you've missed a pill, quite another realizing you've missed two in a row just as the body on top of you is rolling off. The likelihood of you falling pregnant is affected by many factors (see below). If you're over sixteen and in doubt, pop down to your local pharmacist and buy the Emergency (Morning After) Pill over the counter. In some countries it may be necessary to visit your doctor for a prescription or to visit Family Planning or Planned Parenthood. At present, you can also buy it over the Net but there's some contention over whether this will continue. You need to take it within seventy-two hours of unprotected inter-course, but the sooner the better. You'll pop two pills within twelve hours and – here's the bad news – they might not be the most pleasant hours of your life. Lots of people feel sick and are sick, as I'm sure you have been after a punishing night out. You need to weigh up what's worse: hangover-type symptoms or an unwanted pregnancy?

- **He withdrew too late:** People scoff at the withdrawal method of contraception but when practised properly, it can be quite a successful means of contraception. If he withdraws every single time and you're experienced at it, it fails about once every four years. Your chances of getting pregnant by him withdrawing too late are the same as the chances of getting pregnant after having sex just once: it's unlikely but not that unlikely. If you're trying to get pregnant, you're told it takes around two years of regular intercourse for the average couple to conceive. If you're trying *not* to get pregnant, you're told it only takes one time. Go figure. It depends on myriad factors, like whether you're ovulating at the time (usually mid-cycle) how old you are, what your fertility history is, the position you choose and whether he's drunk so much his sperm haven't got a hope of swimming to the side of the pool, let alone doing a whole length. If you're worried, get the Emergency Pill.

- **Everything just went wrong:** The condom broke or slid off, your diaphragm got knocked out of place, you can't find the strings of your IUD or you're overdue for your Depo-Provera shot: all of these put you at risk and if getting pregnant is about as welcome as the Grim Reaper offering to share a cab, get the Emergency Pill. Yes, you'd have to be pretty unlucky to get pregnant from one slip-up but it's a life-changing slip-up if it does happen. You can get a termination (abortion), but it's an unpleasant form of emergency contraception with possible side-effects. If the contraception that failed was a barrier method, it also means you might have to consider getting an STI/HIV test. More on than that scary topic . . .

You have several options on how to cope with this alarming information: never have sex again, have sex without performing any risky activities (that'll be phone sex, then) or protect yourselves as best you can within a relationship. While the only real protection against STIs is celibacy, the second best is having a monogamous relationship, when both of you have been tested for STIs and given the all-clear. In that situation it's relatively safe to ditch the condoms, but this, of course, only applies if both of you are faithful. If you don't entirely trust your partner, keep using them or book in for a regular STI check-up once a year or every six months. If you're not in a monogamous relationship but sexually active, be as sensible as you can be. Do a visual check for any outward symptoms – sores, blisters, discharge, rash, redness – use a condom with lubricant for all penetrative sex (good quality and correctly used). Don't swallow during oral sex, don't 'rim' without some barrier between you and their anus (cut up a condom) and, if you're really serious about this, put a piece of cling film between you and the person's genitals when performing oral sex. Book in for a test – Google 'sexual health clinic' in your area – once or twice a year and get a *full* test. This will include not just a blood test but urine test, throat swab, pap smear and genital swab. And yes, it's not pleasant getting a long cotton bud inserted into your urethra guys, but it's only for two or three seconds. Ask to be tested for HIV/AIDS, HPV, syphilis, hepatitis B, chlamydia, gonorrhoea and herpes simplex virus 2.

It sounds, and is, a pain to do, but once you've been tested a weird thing happens: you get the all-clear and all of a sudden get the urge to be a bit more responsible. You've got away with it so far (even the least anxious ➢

feel a sense of relief when the results are negative) and now there's incentive to be careful in future.

By the way, the answer to the question of 'How do you know if your partner has been tested or not?' is this: you could go with them if you don't trust them, though if you don't trust them to do this, it's unlikely they'll be faithful anyway, which makes the trip kind of pointless. Or you could ask them what it was like getting tested. If a guy doesn't launch into a detailed ohmigod-type description which revolves around that long cotton bud thing, there's a fair chance he went to the pub instead. Women, bless us, tend not to lie about things like this. We've been having pap smears for years, so it all feels like less of a big deal.

Why am I desperate for sex when I'm single, then desperate to avoid it once I'm in a relationship?

Because we're human and fickle, always wanting what we can't have, and because we gorge ourselves in the early stages of a relationship, then tend to follow it with a sexual starvation regime. Sex goes in stages. In the beginning, abstinence and raw lust make anything feel good, so we enthusiastically shag away, without too much thought as to what we're doing. Then just when the novelty starts to wear off, real life kicks in – ignored, sulky friends and annoyed bosses – and sex takes a back seat. What happens after that is crucial. Early sex is fuelled by passion, a brilliant smokescreen for bad technique or a selfish attitude, while long-term sex is fuelled by technique, imagination and effort. Once the 'newness' wears off, your libidos plummet and you have to work at turning yourself and each other on because desire is no longer automatic. Taking a head-in-the-sand approach guarantees you'll both be bored senseless within a year.

While it's not possible to have great sex all the time – even couples who rate their sex life as fantastic admit only two or three sessions out of every ten are shred-the-sheets stuff – it is possible to have good, satisfying sex most of the time. If you're not and you truly do put the effort in, the chances are you've picked the wrong person. While it's extremely sensible to choose a long-term partner for non-sexual reasons (they're honest and faithful) hitching up with someone you don't fancy isn't (you won't be).

2 How Good Are You In Bed?

And how to be much, much better

••

You've never had any complaints but . . . how does anyone *really* know how they rate on the great-in-bed scale? After all, those groans and moans may well have been staged, your lover's rapturous ravings inspired by love not lust and repeat performances demanded because of a desire for sex, rather than sex with you in particular. Do we ever really know whether that quirky little sex move wows, or if our lovers are simply too embarrassed to tell us it's rubbish because *we're* so chuffed with it. In short, is there a way to find out if sex with us lives up to feverish expectation or provokes bitter disappointment? Are our lovers finally getting to ride in the front seat of that spanking new Porsche, only to find out the plush leather seats are actually vinyl, there's no CD player and the car putters along at 30mph?

I think there *are* ways to tell how you rate as a lover, they just have nothing to do with things like how many partners you've had or how many orgasms you've dispensed. Being a terrific lover isn't about winning some type of sex 'contest', scoring points against your partner or 'bigging' yourself up, being great in bed is about knowledge, practice and attitude. Technique is obviously important (see Chapters 3 and 4 for practical and specific guides), but it's not pivotal because what works for one, won't work for all.

The way to truly find out how you rate as a lover and, more importantly, put yourself on the path to being the best lover you can possibly be, is to first establish how much you know about sex and identify any mistakes you may be making.

Once that's done you can focus on your attitude to sex. By looking at the messages you got from your parents, and other influences, you'll be able to challenge any beliefs that stop you feeling relaxed and uninhibited in bed. Add a number of devious tips and tricks designed to instantly impress and you're well on your way to 'God, you're good!' post-coital compliments.

THE SEX MISTAKES PEOPLE MAKE MOST OFTEN

The first step to finding out what sort of lover you are is to check you're not committing any of the following common carnal sins. Are you guilty of any (please don't tell me all) of the following?

The mistakes men make

- **Men think they have a stronger sex drive than women:** Wrong. The reason why men remain the main sexual instigators, isn't just to do with desire, other factors have a big influence. Women are more likely to do the housework on top of holding down a job: result – we're more tired. Hormones influence our libido: result – we're likely to feel like lots of sex at a particular time, rather than all of the time. Women also tend to attach more emotions to sex: result – if you're being a right so-and-so out of bed, we aren't going to want to jump in one with you. Finally, there's evidence that while men are aroused by the *thought* of sex, women are more aroused by *sensation*. This basically means we might be a bit lacklustre at the start, but we'll heat up nicely once things get going.

- **Men think women want loving sex rather than lusty sex:** I can see how you might be getting confused with this one because we do give a few conflicting messages. Most women need you to touch their clitoris gently with your fingers and tongue, especially at the start. Because of this gently-does-it approach, you assume passionate, lusty thrusting is also out of bounds, not to mention throwing her up against a wall, ripping her knickers off with one hand and, rather forcefully, massaging a breast with the other. Well, the two *aren't* mutually exclusive. While we like a soft touch in some places, we're not adverse to a bit of rough handling of other parts. The trick, as with everything to do with sex, is to ask what she feels like generally as well as on that particular day. It's got a lot to do with hormones and all that girly stuff you don't completely understand (neither do we, by the way). And, of course, it also depends on the individual. I have to generalize in order to give you some sort of guideline, but while *most* women like a gentle clitoral touch, others like it hard, fast and furious. Some women even like it if you nip and bite their clitoris – but proceed with caution and note the word 'some' – it's not usual.

- **Men think women aren't as 'dirty' as they are:** Think you're the only one conjuring up lurid, graphic fantasies about other passengers on the tube? Think again. That girl you're sneaking looks at could well be doing the same thing. In a recent study which measured blood flow in the genitals (blood flow increases when we're turned on) women turned out to be more aroused by explicit fantasies than romantic ones. We aren't the dainty, effete creatures you think we are. If you don't believe me, flick through a

Nancy Friday book about female fantasies next time you're browsing the book stores. She got women worldwide to send her their personal favourites, and believe me they aren't about men on white horses and romantic walks along the beach!

- **Some men still cling to the myth that women orgasm purely through intercourse:** I'm not going to harp on about this one because it's mentioned about five billion times in this book, but only 30 per cent of women can climax from penetration alone. Most need stimulation of the clitoris by hand or vibrator during intercourse, or for you to perform oral sex or hand stimulation before or after intercourse, in order to orgasm. It's not your fault or her fault that your penis isn't enough; it's a design fault in the female body. The clitoris is *outside* the vagina, rather than inside it – not terribly helpful of whoever has the female body patent, I agree. True, some women claim to have fabulous orgasms through front vaginal wall stimulation, but the good old-fashioned clitoral orgasm is far more common and reliable.

Another good reason to pull on a condom: it could block a virus which causes cancer. Scientists now have proof that condoms prevent the spread of human papilloma virus which causes cervical cancer. The study followed eighty-two women over three years and found that those who always used condoms were 70 per cent less likely to become infected with HPV than those who didn't.

- **Men think all women want big penises:** I'm not going to lie to you, the majority of women *would* prefer to unbutton those sexy jeans of yours and wrap an eager hand around an average, or slightly bigger than average penis. 'I just love an undersize penis!' doesn't often make it on those 'Top five things women want from a man' lists in magazines, but then again neither does an enormous one. The vast majority of women *do not* want large penises. Read that sentence three times, then repeat after me, 'Women do not want large penises.' Unless, of course, you have a large penis, in which case, change it to, 'Women don't just want me because I have a large penis.'

If anything, width tends to count more than length. This is because nearly all the nerves of the vagina are concentrated in the first inch or so and a thicker penis connects with more nerve endings, so can feel more satisfying. The vagina 'balloons' when aroused, so while a long penis reaches further, it's not as tight up that end as it is near the vaginal entrance. All this really is irrelevant, though, because by assuming the size of your penis is crucial, you're placing too much emphasis on penetration. As I said earlier, she's more likely to have her orgasms via your tongue, fingers or a vibrator. It's not that women don't love intercourse just as much as you do (well, nearly as much) it's just not the be-all and end-all. This is supposed to make you relaxed not depressed by the way.

It's under duress that I'm going to give you the measurement of an 'average' penis. I know if I don't you'll end up manically searching the net and God knows what you'll come up with, and at least this way you'll get accurate information. Measure the side of the penis facing your stomach. Put a cloth measuring tape at the base, where it joins your abdomen and measure the distance from there to the top. Erect, the average penis is 5–7 inches long (13–18cm) and three inches (8cm) flaccid (not erect). It's about five inches (13cm) in circumference (that's *all* the way around, not measuring side to side, by the way). Now, let's move away from the penis-size issue, guys – that's right, nothing to see here – and onto other more important stuff, like . . .

- **Men think sex isn't sex without intercourse:** It's your main course with foreplay as the starter. For lots of women, foreplay is the main course and intercourse is a rather delicious side order. Get in the habit of being specific when you talk about sex. Divide it up: say, oral sex, hand stimulation, intercourse. This reinforces the idea that sex is about a lot more than penetration, and it stops you being penetration focused. Let's be honest here: if all you're interested in is sticking your bit inside our bit, the whole bloody thing would be over in minutes every single time. Not even you want that, surely? Think of sex as giving and receiving pleasure and it can last indefinitely.

- **Men think women are impressed if they change positions lots during intercourse:** It's always wise to mix things up a bit, but don't do it purely for the sake of it, especially at the start. Changing positions works best when you know each other's orgasm patterns because you can sense when the other needs more stimulation or is close to climaxing and choose a position to suit. Showcase every position you know in one session simply to show off and you seriously won't want to hear what she'll be telling her friends over coffee the next day. (Yawn!)

- **Men worry if they don't give a woman at least one orgasm:** Excellent news! Oops, sorry, I'm not supposed to say that, am I? Except after centuries of the scales being tipped the other way, it's rather nice to have you all fussing about, asking 'What can I do?' and 'Is this right?' and generally getting het up about it.

Previously, men tended to think of women as sweet, passive lie-back-and-think-of-England types, but now we've morphed into demanding, sex-mad beasts who are inclined to say 'Off with his head!' if you don't deliver an orgasm. But while this, bizarrely, does show progress, the whole thing's been misconstrued. It's great to take her needs into account but don't rate each sex session as 'pass' or 'fail' based on how many times she climaxes. This brings us right back to square one: orgasm-focused sex. First it was yours, now it's hers.

Another reason not to judge your performance on our climaxes is that it's much harder to bring a woman to orgasm than a man, especially if you don't know her body well. Plenty of women don't have regular orgasms with their regular partner ever, so it's highly unlikely she's going to have one the first time you have sex with her. If she knows that not having one is going to dent your confidence, she's liable to fake it and *whoosh!* we've just slid back another dozen years. Sex *is* better with an orgasm thrown in but it's still damn good if it doesn't happen. Think of sex as a journey not a destination.

- **Men tend to rush women to orgasm:** The single, biggest mistake even experienced male lovers make is to underestimate how long women take to orgasm. The statistic most cited for oral sex – the fastest, most direct route – is twenty minutes from first lick to last shudder. That gives you a bit of an idea, but it also depends on how turned on we were before you even touched us, what's being done to us, who's doing it and how much we've had to drink (two drinks and it's delayed, over four and forget it, everything's numb!) What's a guy supposed to do? Well, stop thinking of oral sex or heavy petting as paying your dues and instead think of them as complete sex acts in themselves. Assume we'll take about twenty minutes, settle in and get into it. Let yourself get turned on by turning her on. If your tongue hurts, relax it, making it nice and wide and let her wiggle against you. If your neck hurts, change position or put pillows under her hips. But don't ever ask if or when she's going to orgasm – you'll know when she's about to or has done.

The mistakes women make

- **Women think men are always ready for and always want sex:** If you're talking about a seventeen-year-old who's just landed his first girlfriend, you're quite right. It's likely he will walk, talk, daydream and want to have sex every waking second (and when he's not as well). But once a man hits his mid-twenties, and often before, other parts of his life start to become equally important and all that energy and focus is needed else-where. Real life dampens a lot of men's sex drives more efficiently than a bucket of water poured over a lit match. Work, stress, pressure, bills, arguments – they all stop him, and you, feeling like sex, all day, every day. He's not like your vibrator, you can't just plug him in and expect him to perform on cue. This is why we own vibrators. There is a man attached to that penis.

> *Millions of men are saying no to sex because an increase in stress means they just don't feel like it. According to a survey by Men's Health Forum, 15 per cent of men polled said mental health problems were badly affecting their sex drive.*

- **Women think sex is over once he ejaculates:** Yes, this is often the case. A selfish or misguided lover will collapse into a heap, say 'That was great,' and leave you dry and sadly not high. But while his penis might be temporarily out of action, there's nothing wrong with his hands or his mouth. What's to stop you saying to him, 'Hey, we're not finished yet' and asking him to stimulate you with his hand. Then, when he's got his breath back, he can move onto giving you oral sex (If he's squeamish, leave 'wet wipes' by the bed or nip to the loo for a quick wash). If his orgasm has wiped him out – and in his defence, his body does get flooded with 'sleepy' hormones immediately after orgasm – explain to him that you need to have yours *before* he does.

- **Women don't realize sex is more than just sex to men:** Men often have sex to feel wanted. Granted, it's hard to accept he's after affection when he has one hand up your jumper and the other diving up your skirt, but that just might be the case. Sex for men appears to be a primal form of giving – it's a way for him to feel accepted both physically and emotionally. Because some men still aren't as verbose or comfortable with expressing emotion as women are, sex tends to be used as a means of showing his love and getting close to you. So, if he really wants to say 'I love you', he may suggest sex. If he feels emasculated at work, sex with you could well make him feel manly again. If he's feeling all vulnerable after a health scare, sex is his way of proving to himself that he doesn't have to go through it alone. All of this means that when you reject sex with him, you're not just rejecting sex. In his eyes, you're effectively saying, 'I don't like or want you.' Adopt a new philosophy: don't say no, say when and always make it clear you're saying no to sex, not a cuddle or cosy chat.

- **Women worry too much about their body during sex:** Putting on two pounds is not grounds for avoiding sex for two weeks. Waiting for a 'thin day' may mean you'll never have sex again, even if you make Kate Moss look hefty. It's a sad fact that most women aren't happy with their bodies. Why and what to do about this is impossible to cover completely here, but if your body image is seriously compromising your sex life, get help. See a counsellor, join a support group or read some reputable self-help books.

If body worries are simply making you self-conscious – you don't like him looking at you naked and avoid certain positions because you'll look fat or less than perfect – you can do something about it *now*. First, give yourself a huge kick up the bottom so you land somewhere in reality, which is this: if a man obviously wants to have sex with you, he thinks you're the sexiest woman on the planet at that moment. If he wants to have sex with you again, he obviously liked your body enough to come back for more, and (shock horror) if you suddenly find you're having sex with the same bloke for months or years on end, it's probably safe to assume that he finds you sexually attractive. It's also worth remembering that lots of men find curvy women *way* more attractive than the skinny girls you envy because they find flesh sexy and sensuous.

> **Men who wear aprons when they cook are twice as likely to have sex in the kitchen. Whether women actually want to bed a man in a 'pinny' is debatable.**

I've resorted to an overly simplified way of explaining this because women (me included, I'm ashamed to say) have become so distorted in their thinking about weight and their body that logic tends to go out the window. Try to accept that *he* thinks you look great and sexy, even if you don't agree, then make a pact to focus on what you're *feeling*, not what you look like, during sex. Close your eyes and keep them shut to begin with, if that helps. You might just find you're not only worrying less about your body, you're enjoying sex more.

- **Women don't give men instructions:** His sexual system is simple. If he wants sex, his penis gets hard, he wiggles it about a bit in a nice, warm snug spot and has an orgasm. It's join-the-dots stuff. Einstein would have had problems figuring out the female sexual system – it's so complicated. If you don't show him or tell him how to touch you – when, where, how hard, how fast, in as much detail as possible – you might as well both give up there and then. But you're not going to do that, are you? Just by buying this book, you're admitting you want good sex, so at the very least, you should earmark a few relevant pages and ask him to read them 'because you're a bit shy to say it out loud'. That's not too hard, is it? Neither is opening your mouth and letting out a little groan to let him know you like something, or giving a one-word command like, 'Softer'. Take baby steps and you'll get there.

- **Women over-react when he suggests trying something new:** If your partner came home and said, 'Do you know what, honey? I've had a chicken sandwich every day for lunch for the past two months, so I might try tuna tomorrow', you would think, *What a boring old fart he is! How the hell did he manage to eat the same thing every day for that long?* In short, you'd think it was totally understandable to try something new, which it is.

    Why then, do most of us become paranoid when our partner dares to suggest a change to their sexual menu? Most couples do the equivalent of eating chicken sandwiches day in, day out, year in, year out by following exactly the same pattern each time they have sex. Wanting change is nothing to feel threatened by. Men, and any sexually healthy female, just like looking at, trying out and experiencing new sexual things. There are no sinister connotations (He's gone off me) and no menacing undertones (He's learned about all this from having an affair). There's nothing to worry about; it's just a simple, human need for variety.

The mistakes both sexes make:

- **If you're a sensible, intelligent person, you should feel comfortable with all aspects of sex:** A quick read of the 'Top Four Sex Saboteurs' (page 59) should set you straight on this one. You can be a perfectly well-adjusted person and still struggle with the messages you received as a child or an experience you had in your past.

- **Good sex is always spontaneous:** Spontaneous sex is usually good sex, but planning a sex session – anticipating it and looking forward to it – makes for pretty good sex as well. Both can be equally rewarding.
- **A truly good lover knows how to please anyone:** It's extremely likely that someone who knows a lot about sex and has had lots of practice is going to be better in bed than an uneducated, inexperienced virgin. Technically, that is. If the uneducated, inexperienced virgin is someone you're desperately in lust/love with, it might be the best sex you've ever had. It's all a matter of perception. If there's one quality a truly great lover would have (along with good technique and exemplary communication, of course), it's the ability to treat every single partner as an individual. What works for Michael might not work for Mark.

SEX SPY: WHO WAS YOUR BEST LOVER AND WHY?

He says:
'She was streets ahead of any other girl I've slept with because she clearly loved sex so much. She was a total hedonist. Her idea of the perfect day was a three-course lunch with tons of wine, an hour's sleep, then sex for the rest of the day and night. She was up for trying every-thing I suggested, but it was the way she responded when I touched, licked or penetrated her that made it so awesome. Her eyes would practically roll back in ecstasy and you could tell she was right there in the moment. Some girls aren't. It's so bloody obvious they're thinking about something else and just putting up with you. She's just as amazing five years on.'
Pete, 28 ➤

'It would have to be the girl who changed my mind on blow-jobs. I'd listen to all the other guys going on and on about how getting head from a girl was the ultimate, but all the blow-jobs I'd had, hadn't done much for me at all. Then I ended up in bed with this girl and she converted me in five minutes. She used her mouth, her hand and her tongue – God knows what she was doing but it was amazing. I'd never experienced anything like it before, and sadly I haven't since, either.'
Mark, 23

She says:

'It was a black guy I slept with. I'd heard black men were great, but I thought it was all to do with the size of their penis. It's not. He treated my body completely differently than anything I'd experienced before. He seemed to know how everything worked and immersed himself in me so it was all about me, not him. He was the only person who has ever made me orgasm and actually ejaculate through front wall stimulation. He even thrust differently: he held me so my pelvis was tight against his and ground himself into me, rather than thrusting in and out. Sadly, he was as dull as could be out of bed, but by God he was good in it.'
Toni, 42

'My best lover was a guy I was with purely for sex. I always tend to have better sex with guys I don't care about that much – I think it's because I'm not afraid to try new things with them. We were fond of each other, but we both knew sex was the reason we were together. He would tell me graphic fantasies about what it would be like if we had another woman in the bed and the running commentary made me orgasm in half the time it took

HOW TO APPEAR BETTER IN BED INSTANTLY!

One of the easiest and quickest ways to impress a lover is to suggest what appears to be a complicated intercourse position. Not only does it make you look confident of your sexual prowess (most of us find it hard enough fumbling our way into the missionary position at the beginning) it can make you look terribly worldly and sophisticated. Note that I said 'appears to be' rather than 'is' and 'can' impress. Some people – usually women – aren't in the slightest bit stirred by innovative positions because they're more interested in what tricks you can do with your tongue or fingers. So if you're a man, get that bit right first.

> *In one survey of women, a man's body odour was rated more important than his appearance. Find this hard to believe? Imagine your favourite sex symbol has extreme bad breath and body odour. Exactly.*

If you're a girl, you need to be aware that taking control of what position you'll assume early on in your sexual relationship, may scare the hell out of a man who's not terribly confident. Other more secure men will be delighted, of course, but I'm just warning you. If you want to play it safe, try making a subtle move in a position he's chosen. 'Digging Deep', simply involves lifting your legs in the missionary position and putting them on his shoulders. By lifting your buttocks invitingly as he guides you into a rear-entry position, you'll appear more active and engaged, without being threatening. I should add that it pains me to have to warn women not to appear too sexually 'in charge' too soon, because we should have progressed a little further in the equality stakes, but sadly we haven't.

There's something else you need to keep in mind when trying to impress with a pose. The position should *look* difficult but actually be easy. Smoothly manipulating your partner into a position which is erotic but comfortable is one thing, getting them to contort into something awkward and unflattering won't score you any points at all.

Also remember to pick a position which suits the stage of your relationship and reflects how comfortable you are together. Of the positions I've detailed below, I certainly wouldn't suggest 'The Sex Squat' or 'Top Bottom' until I knew, without question, that the woman I was with was comfortable with her body. Actually, given that most women aren't, I'd also wait until she's having a thin day and has had two glasses of wine. If in doubt, always err on the conservative side and work up from there.

Despite the thousands of variations, there are really only five positions for intercourse. Here I've suggested twists on the original which will make you look good but are easy to do.

🄵 FOR HER

Digging Deep (man on top)

It's a subtle variation on the missionary position, but if you're both fans of deep penetration and enthusiastic, unabandoned thrusting, you can't beat it. The top half of your body can't move much but you can make up for it by moving your pelvis both up and down and side to side.

Get into position by: You lie back on the bed, with your top half and bottom on the bed, legs resting on the floor. He penetrates you, then bend your knees back towards your stomach while he supports himself on his hands and thrusts forwards. It's best if he keeps one of his legs on the floor for support and the other on the bed for balance. If it still doesn't feel like he's penetrated deeply enough (who's a greedy girl then?) you can pull your knees even further back and rest your calves on his shoulders or (show-off!) demonstrate how handy that Pilates class was by crossing your ankles behind his neck. Add extra *frisson* by holding your hands above your head to give the illusion you're tied up – better still, get him to actually do it!

Ⓜ FOR HIM

Top Bottom (woman on top)

Don't attempt this one until you're ready to orgasm, because orgasm you will – rather rapidly. This position is extra-stimulating for any guy who likes looking at bottoms (are there any of you who don't?) and for her if she's into anal play. It puts you in the perfect position to gently insert a well-lubricated finger into her anus during intercourse so she gets the delicious sensation of feeling completely 'filled up'. Tons of women love this, but it's not something most couples do in the beginning, so save this little trick for a bit later! Visually, it's stunning – you get a rarely afforded, intimate view of her bottom and genitals. She might think *Gross!* but you'll think, *Great!* She'll like it because it feels naughty and abandoned knowing you're looking at a *very* private area. All round primal, erotic and well worth getting worked up about.

Get into position by: You need a chair for this one and it's best if it's sturdy, with no arms. You sit on it in the usual manner while she goes on all fours in front of you, facing *away* from you. You then pull her towards you, lifting her legs up to wrap them around your waist. She supports herself on her hands as you penetrate. With your hands on her buttocks, move her back and forth to thrust rather than moving your own pelvis (I'm not suggesting you be lazy, you just won't be able to move much). This position looks damn impressive but it's actually dead easy to do.

ⓕ FOR HER

The Sex Squat (rear entry)

Urgent, animal and aggressive, most couples use rear-entry positions when you're both massively turned on. He can thrust more powerfully here than in any other position and while some women flinch at the thought (Ouch! You just hit my cervix!) most are huge fans. Because you can't see each other, it's great for fantasizing later on (better to be unfaithful in your head than actually do it in your bed) and although it looks energetic, you can respond as little or as much as you like. Up the lust level by doing it in front of a mirror and vary it by alternating between leaning forward on your forearms and sitting up straight, leaning back and letting him kiss your neck.

If you like anterior (front) wall stimulation (think the bit under your belly), you'll adore the sex squat. It's ideal for a G-spot-induced orgasm because the penis rubs up directly against the front wall of the vagina. Maximize your chances of this happening by not rushing it and getting him to keep thrusting deep but slow.

Get into position by: You need a chair for this one as well and it's even more important that it's sturdy. If you can, secure it against something or put it near a table or window ledge (it's a good idea to draw the curtains while you're there, too) which he can grab onto to keep things steady. You're going to be precariously balanced and it's very easy to get carried away and find the earth really has moved and you've both crashed to the floor. Not sexy. Ready? OK, you stand on the chair facing away from him, then get in a squatting position, with your hands on the back of the chair for support. He puts his hands on your waist or clasps the top of your thighs (no, he's not simultaneously checking for cellulite) and penetrates gently. It may help if he puts one leg on the chair to keep it steady while leaving the other on the floor. As I said, keep it *slow*. Move your bottom from side to side for a unique, intense sensation.

Ⓜ FOR HIM

The Sideways Swoon (side entry)

I always think of side-entry sex as Sunday Morning Sex: lazy, relaxed and literally laid back. After all, you really can only do this one lying down! While it lacks the urgency or deep penetration of other positions, side-entry sex features on most couples' favourites list simply because the starting position,

> **The pleasure women get from connecting via words gives the biggest neurological reward you can get outside of orgasm.**

spooning, is how lots of couples tend to sleep. And if you're going to bed or waking up a little horny, it seems like the most natural thing in the world to take advantage. Your bits are against her bottom, which is so close to other inviting parts and . . . Gosh! How did that happen?

Get into position by: You both lie on your sides and get into the classic spoon position, with you curled into her lower back. You enter from behind to assume the traditional side-entry sex position. She then brings her knees up to her chest, altering both the penetration and angle of entry to make things nice and tight. You mould yourself into her so you both end up in an almost foetal position – while having very grown-up fun! Another easy way to alter side-entry sex is to try a different leg position. Get her to lie on her side, but instead of having her legs straight, get her to lift one up towards the ceiling. Tell her to think of the leg lifts she does at the gym: one leg on the floor, the other high in the air. You enter, keeping your legs *between* hers, which are parted as wide as she can get them. As you're thrusting, you're in the perfect position to reach around with your hand and stimulate her clitoris – how handy!

F FOR HER

Reverse Wall Thrust (standing)

Standing positions aren't the most comfortable, which is probably why they work best for quickies. Most of us have sex standing up when we're dying for it, feeling particularly energetic or need to have sex in a hurry, (having it somewhere we shouldn't or with someone we shouldn't be with). It's not ideal for bringing you to orgasm in the usual way – consistent, unhurried clitoral stimulation is awkward and sometimes impossible standing up – but the urgency and thrill factor can often push you over the edge into orgasmic bliss. Also, in most cases you can simply drop to the floor or onto a bed without changing position if you both get weary.

Get into position by: The usual position has you standing with your back against a wall, him lifting you up and supporting you by putting his hands on your buttocks, then bouncing you up and down. For the reverse wall thrust, he enters you from behind as you stand and lean towards a wall, bending over so he can penetrate, then pressing hard against it for support. By simply turning around, you're making it far less strenuous. Not only that, he can thrust harder while you push back with your buttocks, making circles or moving from side to side. Keep your feet on the floor and lift your bottom up, or bend your knees to adjust the height difference.

SIMPLE TRICKS TO IMPRESS

Other little tricks to stand out from the rest and score sexual Brownie points.

Ⓜ FOR HIM

- Adjust your thrusting style. Don't just move in and out, try moving sideways. Or try grinding in a circular motion, keeping the pressure on the clitoral area by maintaining contact throughout.
- During the standard rear-entry position – her on all fours, you behind – put your knees on either side of her instead of kneeling between her legs. In this position you can move forward so you're 'riding her', virtually sitting astride her back. While it's obviously not for tall/tiny combos, it's actually very sexy and not uncomfortable for her at all. ➣

THE PASSION ASSASSINS

We live in a society that bombards us with information about sex. A small portion of it is accurate and useful, the rest gives us false expectations, muddles our mind and makes us feel guilty or ashamed about perfectly normal sexual urges. How good you are in bed is more influenced by the messages your mind tells you about sex than anything else. We aren't born with an attitude to sex, we learn it. 'It's passed onto you by your parents, branded on your brain by your teachers and preachers, carved into your heart by friends and lovers and broadcast to you by the media. Throughout life and on an ongoing basis, these forces continually mould your attitude to sex,' say Michael Broder and Arlene Goldman, the authors of *Secrets of Sexual Ecstasy*. And if that statement didn't scare the hell out of you, it should have.

You've probably heard experts name the brain as our body's biggest erogenous zone. This is a phenomenal understatement. Your mind is so incredibly powerful: it not only controls how you feel about sex, it's almost totally responsible for what sort of sex life you have. If you want to be the best lover you can possibly be, you need to be aware of any sexual beliefs or values which may be adversely affecting how you behave in bed.

Our mind starts collecting messages about sex the minute

our brain starts to process our thoughts. Rather sensibly, most of us re-examine the things we've been told as we get older. If you went to a strict, religious school and got told sex was something to be endured rather than enjoyed, the chances are you challenged and changed this belief once you had a steady sexual partner. For a lot of people, women especially, we're able to change our sexual belief system intellectually but the old belief stays with us emotionally. 'Even though I know it's OK for women to have casual sex, I still feel like I've been used or slutty if it doesn't turn into a full-on relationship and I'm forced to see the guy again,' says my friend Rowan, ruefully. Outdated or inaccurate values act as stop signs in bed. They stop us trying new things and experiencing pleasure guilt-free, and any sex therapist will tell you that giving yourself permission to enjoy sex is a crucial component of having a great sex life.

> **Don't let a guy hug you if you don't want to trust him. Research shows the female brain naturally releases oxytocin after a twenty-second hug, bonding her to the person and triggering the brain's trust circuits.**

This section of the chapter looks at people who may be influencing your sex life and talks about how to break free of harmful beliefs. Granted, challenging your belief system isn't half as much fun as trying out a new sex trick or position, but if the pay-off is a radically revolutionized sex life, I'd say that's worth the effort, wouldn't you?

THE TOP FOUR SEX SABOTEURS

Your Ex: They don't just bugger off with half your photos and DVD collection, lots of exes change the way we feel about sex and our body for ever. Sometimes this is a good thing. If your ex made you feel more fancied than an eighteen-year-old big-breasted blonde popping out of a cake at a sixty-year-old's birthday party and enthusiastically embraced everything you did in bed, you're in nice shape, and probably raring to go for your next lover. If they criticized your sexual performance or appearance and generally made you feel awful about yourself, you're probably hoping you never have sex again. But hold off before posting that application for a job as a lighthouse keeper, because it is possible to undo the damage they've done.

If you had good sexual relationships with other exes, make a list of every nice thing they told you. Compare this list to a list of what the not so complimentary ex said. See how silly their comments seem now? If you're good friends with any of your exes, tell them what happened and ask them to give an honest opinion. Consider the critical ex's agenda: did all this happen *after* he/she suspected you might leave? If so, dismiss it – it's simply sour grapes. If they were insecure or jealous, they may have put you down to make you feel insecure so you'd be less likely to leave them. Finally, if you think your ex actually had a point about some things, read this section carefully, invest in a few other good, informative and instructional sex books and if you get stuck, take yourself off for one or two sessions with a reputable counsellor or sex therapist.

The stars of your favourite TV show: Even if, intellectually, we know life isn't like the soaps or TV series we're addicted to, if you tune in often enough your subconscious starts to believe it is, and you start to feel a niggling sense of sexual dissatisfaction, secretly worrying you don't measure up. Well I'm here to tell you I'm damn *sure* you don't measure up – no-one does, not even the actor or actress playing the part. TV sex isn't real sex, it's not even close to it. Even when the writers attempt to take responsibility for brainwashing millions and throw in a mildly plausible sex problem, it's either blown out of all proportion or solved within five minutes. Remind yourself before you turn on the TV, and when you turn it off: these people aren't real so I can't compare myself to them.

Your friends: Trusted and sexually knowledgeable friends can be invaluable sources for checking if something is 'normal' or not, but you need to be acutely aware that the information they give you could be a slightly altered version of the truth. Research shows that people tend to over-exaggerate the positives of their sex lives when we first meet them, trying to make themselves look good. Once we're fast friends, we tend to over-exaggerate the downside, so as not to make our friends feels inferior. If there's a bit of competition between you, that innocent chat about sex could turn into an opportunity for them to score points; if your friend's too nice, you'll also get misinformation because she'll try to protect you. If you're really worried about something, look it up in a good, reliable sex book before asking a friend's opinion. Be wary of checking on the net. While some sites are brilliant (see 'Useful Contacts', pages 288–91) a lot of it is boastful rubbish eagerly typed in by someone who knows no more about sex than your five-year-old niece.

Your family: The genes you inherit influence your personality, relationships with other people and your sex drive. If Mum or Dad had a high or low libido, there's a good chance you do too. We're all products of the generation before and your parents' attitude to sex heavily influences what you'll think about it. If you grew up with parents who shuddered at the sight of bare knees and still stuck to the stork story when you were twenty, your sexual blueprint will obviously be different from someone whose parents walked naked around the house and sent them off on dates with handfuls of condoms. Even if you end up with strongly opposing views, which often happens if your parent's attitude to sex was extreme, you're still reacting to their initial viewpoint.

How your mother and father relate to each other sexually also has an effect. As much as the thought of our parents having sex makes most teenagers want to curl up and die, we secretly quite like to think they do it occasionally. As teenagers we're sponges, soaking up everything we can glean about sex, our sexual antennae on permanent alert. Did your Mum and Dad have a habit of disappearing mysteriously for 'afternoon kips' after their boozy Sunday lunches with friends? From that you'd get the message that sex is a pleasurable, recreational weekend activity, that alcohol stimulates our sex drive and that it's not socially acceptable to come right out and say, 'Right then, we're off for a quick shag'. If your experience was radically different and you watched your mother freeze whenever your father showed any affection, you learned that sex was something that caused tension and embarrassment.

Our parents' influence on our attitude to sex is so important that it's likely you still carry some of the beliefs they taught you into the bedroom today. As you'll find out when you continue reading . . .

ARE YOUR PARENTS GETTING IN BED WITH YOU?

There are several keys areas which your parents and upbringing may have influenced heavily. I'm going to deal with each of them individually but you'll also find general tips on getting rid of negative sex beliefs on pages 67–8 (Break Free of Bad Beliefs).

You feel uncomfortable touching or being touched:

If touching makes you feel awkward, it could be because you've been touched inappropriately as a child (if you suspect this, you might consider making an appointment to see a therapist to talk things through) or it could be because your parents weren't terribly touchy-feely. It's also likely you're having problems with sex, since it's impossible to have sex without touching.

One of the most vivid moments of my life was watching a man who hadn't been touched in a very long time, receive a hand and shoulder massage. His name was John and I was helping him improve his chances of finding love for a TV show called *Would Like to Meet*. John was forty, a virgin and, while terribly charming and clever, he had virtually no relationship skills. He told me his parents rarely touched him as a child and had never expressed affection, so I thought a massage would help get him used to other people touching him. It took a good hour to persuade John to do the exercise and he agreed to have it only through his clothes – he couldn't cope with being directly touched on his skin – but it was a pivotal point of change. 'I was touched more in that last twenty minutes than I have been in twenty years,' John said afterwards. This simple, sad statement suggested just how deep the touch/trust issue ran. To confront it, I got John do a 'bodymap', a brilliant exercise devised by Aline Zoldbrod (and if you're struggling with childhood issues, I'd strongly suggest you read her book, *Sex Smart: How Your Childhood Shaped Your Sexual Life and What to Do About It*). To make a bodymap you simply draw a rough picture of the outline of your body, then colour it in with different coloured crayons. Each colour corresponds to how comfortable you are being touched in that particular area when you're with – or imagine you're with – a romantic partner in a safe place. A sexually healthy person's body usually ends up mainly green, which means 'I always like being touched here', with some small sections of blue – 'I may or may not like being touched here, it depends on the situation and how I feel' – and tiny sections of red – 'Don't ever touch me there'. John's bodymap was almost entirely red. After several massages and lots of talking, he finally got to experience touch as a pleasant exercise and, I'm desperately happy to report, continues to do so, as he's happily married with a very pregnant wife!

Ways to fix it:

- **Draw your own bodymap:** Think back to your childhood to explain any large red no-go areas which don't appear to be taboo for other people, like our forearms. If you're not happy with the result but aren't sure how to change things, consider visiting a therapist or counsellor.

- **Look at old family snapshots and study the body language:** How close are you all standing? Is anyone hugging or touching each other? Or are you standing stiffly with arms glued to your sides, a safe pace away? Understanding that you feel odd about touch because of your upbringing is the first step to fixing the problem.
- **Start getting regular massages or facials:** Get yourself used to being touched if you're single. Join a dance class.
- **Get a pet:** Stroking a cat or dog is an excellent way to discover how pleasurable it can be to touch, and how pleasurable touch can feel. Animals have no qualms about showing you exactly how much they love it, wanton creatures that they are. They'll press against your hand or leg for more, rudely nudge you to continue, then make happy snuffles or purrs of contentment if you indulge them. If only humans would be as open and honest.

You find it hard to trust partners:

Trust, or the lack of it, is often at the core of sexual dysfunction. Can't get turned on? Having erection problems? Pain on intercourse? Can't really understand what all the fuss is about where sex is concerned? All these feelings could be caused by not completely trusting your partner. In order to trust people, we have to assume that loved ones are worthy of trust. If, like me, you come from a family where one of your parents had an affair, you've learned this isn't necessarily true. Similarly, if one of your parents was an alcoholic, you may have met their needs rather than the other way around. In order to trust our parents, they had to give us consistent, loving attention as a child. If this didn't happen, you don't trust others because you haven't had a positive experience to show you how to.

Other people grew up trusting, but learned not to trust later in life. A cheating partner, a lover who betrays you or runs off with your best friend can all influence our trust systems and leave sexual scars.

Ways to fix it:

- **Get professional help:** How fresh do your trust 'wounds' feel? If you still feel upset and raw thinking about what happened to breach your trust, it's well worth seeing a counsellor. Yes, you could solve it yourself with lots of introspection, soul-searching and a billion self-help books, but a talented, qualified counsellor, psychologist or sex therapist could fix you in a couple of sessions.

- **Isolate the core issues:** Do this if you feel it's not serious enough to seek professional help. What's the scary thing about trusting people? What's the worst that could happen if you did and it turned out to be a mistake? Try to pinpoint particular incidents in your past which have made you feel this way, then focus on people who *have* proved trustworthy and challenge your beliefs. Write things down, putting the 'bad' people on one side of the page, the 'good' people on the other. Zoldbrod also recommends creating 'safe places' – both physical and mental. Meditation and/or hypnosis work, as does a room which is yours only, where you can relax totally and feel safe.

> **Around one-third of girls and two-thirds of boys have masturbated by age thirteen.**

You don't really feel comfortable with anything but 'standard' sex and wouldn't dream of masturbating

Therapists call this not 'giving yourself permission' to explore yourself and your sexuality. To you, it means you're not exactly jumping up and down with excitement when your partner suggests doing something new in bed. In fact, you probably feel more like hiding under it. Again, this is most likely the fault of your parents because very few are interested in or capable of giving appropriate sex education.

Even the most liberal parents get a little tongue-tied and flustered talking about 'rude' or intimate things with their kids. Religious parents may only believe in sex for procreation and ban you from talking about it at all, as well as dispensing dire predictions about what will happen if you touch yourself. My favourite has to be the one that says you'll go blind if you masturbate – charming! Parents who are super-conscious of trying to arm you with all the facts can sometimes go too far the other way and overwhelm and embarrass with too much info too soon. Teenagers need the facts, delivered non-judgementally, but they also need to have their modesty and privacy respected.

Ways to fix it:

- **Write down the three main messages you got from your parents about sex.** What's your reaction to what you've written? Do you still agree with these views now? If so, do you think people you know and trust appear to hold the same views, i.e. do they seem reasonable? If you took one look and burst out laughing at how silly those messages were, it's a good sign that you've moved on without too much damage. If you feel anxious or uncomfortable even seeing the messages written down, and if your sex life leaves a lot to be desired, I would consider seeing a sex therapist. As I said earlier, and will no doubt say again, I'm not suggesting you can't sort it out yourself by reading some good self-help books or talking to friends, but if you're after a quicker, efficient, longer-lasting fix, a good sex therapist is your best bet. Choose one who is accredited and a member of the regulating society or association in your country and talk to them on the phone first to ensure you feel confident they're qualified (see the 'Useful Contacts' list on pages 288–91).

BREAK FREE OF BAD BELIEFS

Are you destined for misery if the people around you weren't exactly sexually inspiring? Not if you recognize the problem and actively set out to break the pattern, say psychologists.

- **Be aware of 'self-talk':** the internal thoughts or dialogue, positive or negative, that play in your mind. These run in a pretty much permanent stream through our minds and are so automatic, we're largely unaware of them. Pay attention and listen to what you're telling yourself.

- **Stop 'spectatoring':** evaluating yourself and your performance during sex, usually negatively. If you're constantly picturing how you look as you're having sex, it not only takes you away from the moment, it makes you self-conscious. Both are desire dampeners.

- **Think about what your values are regarding sex:** are they helping or hindering your sex life? If they're not doing you any favours, ditch them. Everyone else's 'shoulds' and 'should nots' don't apply to you – it's your sex life, not someone else's! Ask yourself, 'If I heard this belief or value for the first time today, would I accept that it's true? Would I want to teach my child this value?' Answer yes and it's your friend. Answer no, and it's your enemy.

- **Actively challenge views you want to change:** write down healthier, alternative messages you'd like to replace the distorted views with, backing them up with as much 'evidence' as possible (see the following points).➢

From this, take the five messages you most want to adopt about sex, pin them to your bedroom mirror and look at them daily. This will help your brain adjust your sexual blueprint.

- **Educate yourself sexually:** Arm yourself with some good sex manuals and start studying. Read the sections that talk about your emotional feelings about sex as well as the technical how-to chapters on improving your love life. The more evidence you have to dispute unhealthy sex messages, the more chance you have of changing them.

- **Work on your self-esteem:** if your experiences have left you seriously doubting your sexual appeal and attractiveness, surround yourself with people who give you confidence or take a few self-esteem-boosting courses to help get you back on track.

F FOR HER:

MODERN SEX MYTHS SHE SHOULDN'T BELIEVE

There are a lot of myths and 'rules' floating about out there, and an awful lot of the ones relating to sex are directed at women. Quite frankly, most are false or misleading. Others reflect an outdated, old-fashioned sexual standard. We might not be totally over the 'men are studs, women are sluts' attitude to sexuality but we're a lot further from it than our parents were. If you're female, do yourself a favour and dismiss most of what you hear. You're better off accepting that some actions are just part of being human. Besides, the fallout often isn't half as bad as you think.

You should never sleep with someone from work

The myth: It's 9.30a.m. on a Friday morning – the morning after a quick one after work turned into a bit of a party for you and a dozen other workmates. They're nursing sore heads and you're trying to pluck up the courage to enter the tea room, wearing exactly what you wore the day before while simultaneously avoiding eye contact with Mike from Accounts. Whoever said you should never mix business with pleasure was right: the embarrassment factor is way too high.

The reality: Two-thirds of us meet our life partners through friends or at work, so why should you be any different? Take refuge in the fact that it's not even your fault because new studies show that close proximity breeds lust. Repeated exposure to practically any stimulus makes us like it more – the only time it doesn't hold true is when our initial reaction to something is negative. When we spend a lot of time with someone, our brain releases attachment hormones, which make us want to hang around pretty much permanently. This actually isn't a bad thing. Couples who meet through work have a much clearer idea of what they're getting themselves into. After all, you've seen your partner react to all sorts of stressful situations during your average working day. As for employer's fears, most are unfounded: what better way to get employees to turn up early,

> ❶ *Trying to bond with a new lover? Forget trading pleasantries – you're better off having a good old bitch! A Texan study found that sharing pet hates or negative opinions can bring people closer together in the beginning than discovering mutual passions. The reason why? It's riskier expressing negative emotion so intimacy builds more quickly.*

stay late, look fantastic, willingly sign up for all extra-curricular activities and generally beam their way through the working day? And even if the affair ends, most flirtations fizzle out with remarkably unspectacular endings, as opposed to the fury of resignations or ruined relations people worry about.

You should always tell the truth about your past

The myth: Around the time you both start going gooey over each other, questions start being asked: 'So . . . who else have you lived with/been out with/been in love with?' If you read the subtitles they clearly say, 'How many people have you slept with?' Even if you've managed to hook up with the world's most liberated guy, few can resist a knee-jerk reaction to an answer of ten or more, mainly because they haven't thought it through. So is it any wonder that you found yourself muttering, 'Three,' and are now panicking about being caught out? But why should you feel bad about having had more than three lovers? A typical thirty-year-old attractive woman has usually been sexually active since the age of sixteen, had two long-term monogamous relationships, each lasting around four years, clocked up two short-term relationships per year the rest of the time and had the odd casual fling. That's around twenty partners, by my estimation, or twenty-five to thirty if you're dealing with a high libido or increased opportunity.

The reality: He's really asking, 'How special am I? Do you behave like this with everyone?' If he's serious about you, he's actually far more interested in what's happened to your heart than your parts, so he won't be obsessed with doing the maths. If he does start doing sums and you are discovered, appeal to his sense of logic. Confronted with the above breakdown and other facts – such as the number of lovers for both men and women is roughly the same these days (although because of double standards men consistently report three times more) most men will see reason. And if he doesn't, is he really the right guy for you?

You should never have sex on a first date

The myth: The phone rings and your best friend's voice chirps cheerfully into the ansaphone, 'Soooooo, how was it? Did you snog him?' You open one eye to see him looking at you to see if you're looking at him. Ohmigod. He's not supposed to be there listening to this. He's not supposed to be in your bed at all.

The reality: I can list at least four couples without even blinking, let alone thinking, who had sex on the first date and are still happily together five or ten years later. If you're old enough, wise enough and have pretty decent people-reading skills, who's to say you can't sum someone up during an average five-hour date, at least enough to know they're worth taking a risk on. Sometimes you just know. And some first dates can be so good, they backfire if you stop the flow. Then there's the pertinent question of what constitutes a first date? If you've been friends for a while and finally go out, are you on date one or date ten? I know I'm being slightly contradictory because I do generally advocate waiting as long as possible, but there are always exceptions.

For truly great sex you should come together

The myth: You've already had one orgasm through oral sex, now he's pounding away and looking at you expectantly, waiting for the signal that number two is approaching so he can let go. He leans down to give you a hand, which sort of works, but you're concentrating so hard on timing your climax to match his that you miss the moment. Now you feel you've got no choice but to resort to faking it.

The reality: Let's take a look at the facts: roughly 75 per cent of men in relationships always have an orgasm with their partner, compared to only 30 per cent of women. Men's orgasms last for around ten to thirteen seconds, women's can last anywhere from twelve seconds to close on two minutes. Do the maths and you'll soon see the chances of both of you orbiting into orgasmic ecstasy at exactly the same moment is unlikely. Soap stars regularly shout 'Yes! Yes! Yes!' in unison, but you'll be hard pressed to find the same scene recreated in bedrooms at home. If you want to up your chances, get him to slow down so you can catch up because women take longer than men to build to the pre-orgasmic phase. Same sex couples could be at an advantage here because their arousal clocks are more in sync.

THE GOOD-IN-BED CHECKLIST

☑ **You're knowledgeable about sex** and have a good understanding of how your body and your partner's body works.

☑ **You've had lots of practice** – it really can perfect your technique.

☑ **You've got the right attitude** – of all these things, attitude – being able to let go and enjoy – is the most crucial.

☑ **You'll try everything (within reason) once** – say, 'I've always wanted to try so-and-so, but I've never felt comfortable enough to suggest it with anyone else before,' you score *huge* points.

☑ **You play games** – the more playful you are in bed, the higher you'll be rated as a lover. Loosen up a little, laugh a lot, drop the inhibitions and let your imagination run wild.

☑ **You initiate sex as much as they do** – it not only feels great their end, it feels good at yours as well. Nothing is more enpowering than being the one undoing the zip and promising the earth in return for having your wicked way.

☑ **You keep your genitals fit** – regular exercise of your PC muscles makes intercourse much better for both of you. The tighter her vagina, the more sensation she'll feel; the more control he has over his PC muscle, the more control he'll have over his erection.

☑ **You spend roughly twice as much time on foreplay as you do on intercourse** – if you've stopped thinking of intercourse as sex and foreplay as the stuff you do before you have intercourse, pat yourself on the back. Get into the habit of having sessions without any intercourse and bring each other to orgasm purely through oral sex or mutual masturbation.

☑ **You put the effort in** – a good lover accepts that great sex doesn't just happen when you're ten years into the relationship.

☑ **You laugh off embarrassment** – if you're not making a fool of yourself now and then, you're staying within your comfort zone. Not good.

☑ **You say no to sex occasionally** – saying yes every single time means you're a 100 per cent Sure Thing. Marriage and living together removes a lot of the chase, so don't wipe out the last shred of it by removing all predictability.

☑ **You know what you want and tell and show your partner** – someone who knows their sexual triggers and isn't afraid to let their partners in on the secret gets the perfect ten.

☑ **Your ex-lovers admit you were great in bed** – if you've stayed friends, the conversation nearly always turns to 'Was I OK? Because you can be honest now'. They might still sugar things up to be nice, but if an ex raves about your past performance between the sheets, it's a safe bet they're telling the truth. If more than three exes adored one particular signature sex move, your sexual esteem gets an extra boost. Knowing you have a guaranteed knee-trembling, moan-maker works wonders.

3 The Nitty-gritty

Hot new techniques to try

● ●

Good sex isn't reliant on good technique, but if you're talking long-term, by God it helps. The clumsiest fumble feels great if it's the first time someone you've salivated over touches you. Inept, incompetent love-making with a lover who's had years to suss out your sexual triggers doesn't. Once lust and newness wear off, our bodies need more experienced handling to get the same result, which is why lots of couples start to hit problems about three months into a relationship.

The person you need to give a talking to, however, isn't necessarily your partner. It's presumed the more sex you have, the more they'll get to know your body and what you do and don't like. But this is only true if *you* show or tell them, or at the very least give heavy hints via body language or groans. With no feedback, they're left fervently hoping it feels all right your end, without ever really knowing. This is why chapters like this, which detail techniques, are included in most sex books.

Sexual technique – how to do something properly – starts

to obsess us from a young age, with most little boys going through a stage of practise kissing Mummy. Once we've passed through the innocent toddler stage, learning sexual technique becomes more difficult (practising on family members being clearly out). While there are lots of sexual references in the media, practical, non-judgemental, easy-to-follow information on technique forms only a tiny part of that. *The Sex Inspectors*, a TV show I did, concentrated a lot on teaching couples techniques because it became painfully apparent that most people really hadn't thought much beyond the basics. I took one of the people we worked with on the show to an ice-cream parlour and got him to demonstrate how he gave his girlfriend oral sex by licking an ice-cream. He looked at it perplexed. 'I part her legs and just dive straight in,' he said, confused. 'I'm not sure *what* I do in there!' When I showed him on the ice-cream how most women like men to use their tongue, he was intrigued. (So, mind you, were the dozen or so other people in the ice-cream parlour, who queued up waiting to be served wondering why two people were being filmed manically licking away.)

Even couples who have communicated about sex and are fairly sure they know what their partners want, benefit from dipping in and out of a sex book for new tips and tricks. Not only do our tastes change, using the same technique over and over loses its appeal quicker than ice-cream melts.

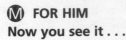 FOR HIM
Now you see it . . .
Just as men's testicles do a disappearing act close to orgasm – the testes need to be retracted for him to orgasm – the clitoris often hides under its hood when she's nearing orgasm. Given that it's a slippery little bugger at the best of times *and* that most men are literally in the dark when

performing oral sex, this can cause more anxiety than running out of beer on the night of the World Cup Final. If this happens to you, don't panic, and don't go looking for it either! Just keep stimulating the general area in which the clitoris was last seen or gently massage her tummy, pressing your palm downward toward the vagina to make it pop back out again.

While we're on the subject of crimes punishable by death, it's *absolutely imperative* that once she starts to orgasm you don't stop stimulating her or change what you're doing. Her orgasm is roughly three times longer than yours and it's common for men to think it's all over when it's only just begun. And here's the thing: while you'll continue to orgasm once you've started, even if she stopped right there and walked out the room to make a cup of tea, women are different. If you stop touching or licking her at the start of her orgasm, it's very likely you'll abort the rest of it and that's about as satisfying as having one bite of a chocolate when you were planning on scoffing the entire box.

SET TONGUES WAGGING
How to give outstanding oral sex

'He's got a small willy,' my girlfriend said over the phone, reporting on her new boyfriend. 'But he's absolutely brilliant at oral sex, and out of the two, I'd have to say that's more important to me.' Hands up those women who agree. While a big penis is indeed a nice bonus, that's just Mother Nature having a generous day. Being able to deliver delicious oral sex has nothing to do with being born with a big tongue, it takes skill, and it says a lot about a person. To be really, really good at giving oral sex, you have to be a generous person who enjoys giving as much as receiving. It's a sex act where enthusiasm is all, being squeamish spoils everything and the willingness to take time is paramount. Get it right and you inspire slavish loyalty, with lust-sick partners looking around worriedly if you so much as lick your lips in view of attractive strangers.

> **Every generation thinks they've invented oral sex but it's been practised on men and women for thousands of years. The Egyptians were particularly avid fans – the reason Egyptian prostitutes wore lipstick was to advertise the fact that they were masters at fellatio.**

Oral sex is also about power – in a win-win type of way. Getting someone to lick your bits puts them in a submissive position which used to be thought of as degrading. Dr Glenn Wilson, a psychologist and expert on human sexual behaviour, tells the story of two oral-sex legends, one involving an empress of the T'ang Dynasty. Wu Hu was said to exert dominance over all visiting foreign officials by making them perform cunnilingus on her. But giving great oral sex can put the giver in a power position as well. According to Wilson, Cleopatra is reputed to have been a master fellator and rumoured to have performed oral sex on 100 Roman soldiers in a single night. Odd that she's remembered more for her haircut and eyebrows given this achievement, but there you go! Breasts, penises, clitorises and vaginas hog the limelight, but the organ that's probably most appreciated is the tongue.

Ⓜ FOR HIM

Get into position

Because lots of women rely on oral sex to provide them with their orgasm and tend to take longer than men to reach one, it's crucial that you choose a comfortable position. Lots of experts recommend you use pillows to achieve this: pop one under her bum to raise her genitals and one under your arms/chest. Making sure you're supported and that your head/neck aren't strained can alter both the angle and pressure of your technique, with brilliant results for both.

Take your pick:

- She lies on her back, you lift her up and put her knees over your shoulders, her weight is on her shoulders with her bottom and torso lifted high into the air.

- She gets down on all fours, and supports her weight on her hands and knees, facing you. You slide underneath her, using pillows to prop you up to the right height to reach her bits.

- She's on all fours supporting her weight on her hands and knees but facing away from you, you lick her from behind.

> 'My friends and I nick-named my ex "the man with the mouth". He was so good at giving oral, he became the benchmark against which we measured all our boyfriends, past, present and future. Guys think it's all about the size of their penis, but it so isn't.'
>
> Sandra, 37

- In the standard position, her lying on the bed, knees bent, you lying between her legs – get her to pull her knees up to her chest to open things up .

- She lies on her side, you're positioned between her thighs so her top leg is around your neck. She holds the fleshy part of the mons (the bit covered by pubic hair) up to expose her clitoris.

- She sits on a chair or on the side of the bed, you kneel between her legs.

- She lowers her genitals onto your face but faces your feet, leaning forward and holding onto your ankles for support. This makes it easier for your tongue to directly hit the clitoris.

- She lies on her back, with her hips on the edge of the bed, feet flat on floor. You kneel between her legs, she then pulls her thighs back to her chest, keeping her legs spread wide apart. If she's into bottom play or pressure on her perineum, this one's perfect.

- She stands with her legs apart, you kneel in front of her while she leans back against a wall.

- **Top choice:** You lie on your back on the bed or floor with your knees bent and feet flat on the floor. She kneels over your face, facing you, her legs wide apart and her vagina over your mouth. She then leans backward onto your knees, leaning on them and letting her head fall back. This not only opens her exceptionally wide, allowing for good penetration with your tongue internally, which some women like along with clitoral stimulation, it also puts her breasts in prime view, making them easy to massage.

Get to work

The only real expert on how and where she wants to be stimulated is your partner, says sex guru Bernie Zilbergeld, and never was there a truer word spoken. She may well shrug and say 'Whatever' in the beginning when you ask her what she wants because she's shy, but you've given her the green light to instruct you later without fear of offending. Before your tongue has even connected, you've already scored major points.

Assuming you've paid attention to everything else in this book, you will have teased, titillated and sexually transfixed her to such a point that she isn't just straining for you to do the business, she's thrusting her pelvis forward impatiently. In other words, I'm taking this from the first lick rather than how to get to it. I'm also assuming some basic experience. If you'd like more info, my first book *Hot Sex: How to Do It* is another good source. The basic rules of giving her great oral are this: keep it wet, slow, gentle and consistent. Slow and steady wins this race.

- **Keep it wet:** Mouths get dry and dry oral sex irritates rather than excites. Keep a glass of water handy or take mini breaks to come back up and kiss for a while. (Tell her your mouth is dry if she looks pissed off!) Another way to generate saliva is to double your tongue back to touch the underside to the top of your mouth and hold it there for a few seconds.

- **Keep it slow, gentle and consistent:** Most women prefer repetition when it comes to oral sex: keeping the same pressure, pace and technique won't brand you boring but brilliant. Again, though, be warned that this is a generalization. It works for most but not all, so always ask and be alert to her body language.

- **Flatten your tongue** rather than use the tip and start with big, slow licks, keeping your tongue wide and flat. Alternate little, fast darting licks with a tenser tongue until you can tell which she likes best. Use one hand to pull up the fleshy part of her mons as this makes it easier to see the clitoris. Also, try moving your head up and down as you're licking because your tongue will tire if it does all the work. Experiment with each side – lots of women like one side of their clitoris stimulated more than the other.

- **Experiment** with what's charmingly called 'tongue-fucking': making your tongue as stiff as possible and pretending it's a penis as you thrust in and out. Though I have to say men tend to get more aroused by this than the women they're doing it to, probably because it's a

> *Approaching the infamous seven-year anniversary and worried it'll be your last? Breathe easy – well, for the next three years anyway. German researchers claim it's actually after ten years that marital happiness hits an all-time low, falling lower than it was before marriage.*

technique which relies on penetration to excite rather than clitoral stimulation.

- **Use your hands:** Just as she uses her hand while fellating you, a lot of the work of cunnilingus can be done with your fingers. Use your tongue solo to begin with, then insert one or two fingers inside her vagina, thrusting in time with your licks. Angle your fingers up, aiming towards her pubic hair, to stimulate the more sensitive front wall of her vagina. Then surreptitiously slide one finger between her inner vaginal lips and lick alongside or around it as you slide up and down between them gently. This intensifies the feeling and it's hard to tell whether the sensation is coming from your tongue or finger. Yes it's cheating, but its definitely the forgivable kind.

- **Settle in:** Act like you've got all day and it will make her orgasm faster. Ironic but true! The more you rush her, the less likely it is to happen. The general consensus is that most women take around twenty minutes to orgasm through oral sex, but that entirely depends on how turned on she was beforehand, the time of the month, how much she's had to drink etc. Sometimes she'll orgasm in three minutes, other times it will take thirty.

- **Look like you're enjoying it:** Make noises – groan, say 'mmmmm'. Pull back, look at her displayed in front of you and say 'Oh God' before diving back enthusiastically.

- **Don't forget other parts:** Reach up to massage her breasts, use both hands to cup and massage her bottom, let her suck one of your fingers, insert a finger into her anus or apply pressure to the opening, hold her hand.

Afterwards

- Tell her how much you love the taste and smell of her genitals. Tell her how kissable/shaggable/pretty her vagina is. We all know it isn't exactly the most attractive body part, but it's worth lying through your teeth. Even the most sexually secure woman gets paranoid sometimes about whether she looks, smells or tastes OK so it's nice to be reassured and even nicer if you lick your fingers with relish after touching her. At the time, she may go, 'Yuck, that's gross,' but secretly she'll be pleased. While we're on the yuck-type topics: there's no need to avoid oral sex if she's having a period. Just get her to insert a fresh tampon and pop the string inside. Pull it back down afterwards, though – it's alarmingly easy to forget it's there.

🅕 FOR HER

Get into position

Comfort is probably less important for you giving him oral sex than vice versa, and this is because once he heads south he'll tend to settle in and take it through to completion (not only do lots of us depend on oral sex for our orgasms, our bits are not as fond of intermittent stimulation) it can take a while to build back up to where we were before. Fellatio for men is often something that preludes intercourse and, if you're very, very good at it, usually doesn't last long for this reason – he's keen not to ejaculate so he can 'save' his erection for penetrative sex. If he does want to orgasm through oral sex, positions where you have good access to his testicles, anus and perineum become more important. To take him through to a glorious finale, you'll need to manipulate more than just his penis. The primary rule for picking positions is that his penis likes to point upwards. Yes it is fascinatingly bendy, but seeing how far you can point it downward before it snaps back up is a lot more fun your end than his.

Take your pick:

- You kneel in front of him as he lies on his back in bed. Take him in your mouth, place your knees wide and use your thigh muscles to hold yourself steady and to allow you to use both hands.

- You lie beside him as he lies on his back on the bed, moving yourself down until your mouth is next to his penis. This is a standard position and usually the first one couples use. It's also one of the least effective: it's awkward, you don't have great access to anything and he can't see what you're doing. Ditch it asap!

- You lie on your back, your head propped up with some pillows. He's kneeling over you on all fours, his penis near your face, weight supported on his hands.

- With oral sex, just like intercourse, you need to take height into account. Use stairs, pillows or pieces of furniture to even things up.

- If he likes looking at your bottom and bits, position yourself in a 69 position by lying on top of him, your head facing his feet.

- If his legs buckle while standing, get him to sit on the side of the bed while you kneel before him, or tell him to lean against a wall.

- **Top choice:** You kneel in front of him while he stands, or you sit on the side of the bed while he stands in front of you. These two positions are superior for good reason: they give a sense that you're worshipping his prized part, which gives you ten out of ten before you've even opened your mouth, and

> **Looks like we're from the same planet after all.** Relationship guru John Gottman set out to find out the key factor which determined how satisfied women were with the sex, romance and passion in their marriage. The answer? 70 per cent said it was the quality of the couple's friendship. When men were asked the same question, guess what 70 per cent of them said? Friendship!

they leave you nicely balanced, which isn't the case when you're lying beside him. You have both hands free to work on his testicles, nipples, anus, perineum, and it puts you completely in control of how deeply you take him into your mouth and where he ejaculates (breasts being handily positioned right in front of him).

Get to work:

As with the oral sex guide written for him to pleasure you, I've cut straight to the chase foreplay wise. The rest of this book has ideas on how to get to this point if you need them. Again, the person who best knows how he likes fellatio is him. Ask him to give you a running commentary/feedback on what feels good and what doesn't.

- **The basic rules:** use your hand as well as your mouth, create decent suction but don't suck, start slow and gentle, work up to faster, firmer action. Remember, most feeling is in the head of the penis, so there's no need to 'deep throat' unless you want to – or swallow, while we're on the topic. So long as you warn him and get him to warn you when it's about to erupt, keep working on him with your hand and allow him to ejaculate somewhere nice, like your breasts or neck, he seriously won't mind. If swallowing is so important to him that he's happy to trade a three-hour massage for each time you do it, give it a go. It's not that bad, promise! The trick is either to swallow quickly or hold it in your mouth till he's done, then politely spit it into a tissue by the bed or excuse yourself and spit it into the sink. It's always a good idea, by the way, to avoid visibly gagging, screwing up your nose or saying, 'Ewwww!' really loudly once you've done it.
- **Make eye contact:** Start by looking him in the eyes and sucking his finger like you're going to be working on other bits, *then* move downwards.

- **Decide on your first move:** Dispense a few 'lollypop' licks, licking up and down the shaft and head while holding the penis steady with your hand, then prepare for the first time you take him into your mouth. Some swear it's most effective if you take as much of him as you can, in one heart-stopping, sensational swoop. Others say it's better to tease, covering the head only, swirling your tongue around, then moving millimetre by millimetre down the shaft. I say both work for different occasions and moods.

- **Relax the muscles in your jaw and neck:** Breathe through your mouth and cover your teeth by either pushing your lips out in an exaggerated pout (best), or pulling them back to cover them (second best). Flicking the head with the tip of your tongue will get him as excited as a man about to walk through the front doors of Ikea on a Sunday. Instead, imagine you're licking an ice-cream and give broad, long, slow, lascivious swishes on the head using a flat tongue.

- **Settle into a rhythm:** Place your hand at the base of his penis and move it up and down in the standard 'fist' motion. Let your mouth follow your hand. Get a good rhythm going then start to twist your hand as it reaches the head to provide extra stimulation. Throw in a swirl of the tongue as you slush it around the join between the head and shaft, paying special attention to the frenulum – the stringy bit of sensitive skin where the head of the penis meets the shaft, on the side facing his testicles.

- **Act like you want to be there:** Make noise. Pull back, admire him, then gobble him up again eagerly. Concentrate on what you're doing. If you find yourself pondering how to solve the world's famine problem, it's time to change technique. Even if he's fond of a particular method, stop to change hands/lick or suck his testicles/ kiss him, so your mouth and hand are temporarily removed. This will stop him becoming desensitized and you bored silly.

- **You have lift-off** when his penis swells and turns a purplish red, his testicles shrink and rise towards his body, he thrusts deeper and faster (or goes still for a few seconds) and his body tenses. Other clues are if he shouts 'Ohmigod, I'm going to come!' or grunts and groans like he's in excessive pain. If you're swallowing, stop stimulation completely when he stops ejaculating or thrusting into your mouth. Hold his penis gently in your mouth for a second or two, then remove it. If you're letting him ejaculate elsewhere, remove your mouth and use your hand to masturbate him, letting go after the last spurts of semen.

Afterwards

- Give his penis a little kiss and lay it reverently on his tummy. By all means go back up for a cuddle and kiss, but don't be offended if he hardly reciprocates or seems in another world for a few minutes (hours). Mother Nature is flooding his body with relaxing, sleepy hormones which make him want to crash. The original purpose was to knock him out completely so he'd get maximum rest in a short period of time and be up and raring to go in record time, ready to make more babies to populate the earth. These days it has no function other than to annoy the hell out of women, given that our bodies are flooded with attachment hormones after sex, which make us want to snuggle and bond.

RUN CIRCLES AROUND HER
Most of us follow the same sequence when we have sex, building in sensation and intensity as we continue, rather like climbing stairs with our orgasm happening on the top ➤

one. Beverly Whipple, a well-known sexologist, believes the female cycle of desire is more circular than linear. Men tend to feel desire before arousal – he'll often have an erection before even kissing or touching – and move predictably and steadily towards orgasm. Women often become aroused and feel desire once the action starts, moving in a more erratic pattern towards climax. To make sex better for both of you, Whipple suggests your focus should be on a circular cycle of pleasure rather than orgasm. A typical sex session for most follows a kiss/touch/oral sex/intercourse pattern. Instead, she suggests a session which runs more like this: cuddling and kissing/intercourse (he orgasms)/tie-up game with manual genital stimulation for her/kissing/oral sex (she orgasms)/intercourse (though not to orgasm for either)/oral sex for him (he orgasms)/intercourse and so on. Well, you could go on if you're not crawling towards the bed for sleep. (You're not doing it in bed are you now?) Make up your own list of things you'd like in your circle and mix things up a bit.

ALL-DAY FOREPLAY:
Sex on the hour, every hour

OK, so it's a little ambitious to cram all this into twenty-four hours, though it would be one hell of a day if you did! The idea behind the all-day sex-play plan isn't actually to get you both sacked or to turn you into slightly deranged sex addicts people cross the street to avoid. It's to get you out of the habit of thinking of sex and foreplay as something you do when you're together, at home, in bed, at 10.24 p.m. on a Friday night (sadly, the average time most couples have sex). Just as most people don't actually meet the love of their lives while they're prancing about in a singles bar, G&T in hand and body poured into an LBD, sex doesn't always have to take place at home on weekend nights. It's entirely possible to think about sex and nurture your sex life at *any* time of the day, not just while you're together, as you'll see!

6 a.m.
- 'Femoral intercourse' is a rather handy solution to the sleepy female/awake-and-horny male syndrome. Originally used as a method of birth control and to preserve virginity, it involves him thrusting his penis between your closed thighs instead of inside your vagina. It's a gentle, non-invasive way to have sex and keeps both of you satisfied. If he places his penis near the top of your thighs so it slides in between your vaginal lips, stimulating the clitoris, sleepy female can rapidly turn into wide-awake-horny female!

7 a.m.
- Dress for work like it's a strip club. Nonchalantly pulling on a supersexy bra and knickers, stockings and suspenders, under unassuming office clothes keeps both of you focused on sex throughout the entire work day. She's reminded of it each time she takes a trip to the loo, he's praying to God it really was done for his benefit alone.

8 a.m.
- Write an erotic note describing how hot your last great sex session was and how excited you are by what he does to you. Slip it inside his wallet so he gets a nice surprise when he's buying lunch. (Best fold it, so it's not the little old lady queueing behind him at Starbucks who discovers just how much you like having your nipples bitten.)

9 a.m.
- Kiss goodbye as you both head off to work. But none of that air-kiss rubbish, I mean a good, thorough, deep delicious

snog to end all snogs. After you've spent several moments exploring each other's mouths, slide south, pull down his zipper/pull up her skirt and spend two minutes giving slow, exquisite oral sex before zipping them up again and pushing them out the front door. Get out of the mindset that all sex sessions have to have a beginning, middle and end.

10 a.m.

- Text your partner one sentence of a fantasy and get them to text back the next line. Keep going back and forth until you've finished the fantasy – or your boss is breathing down your neck. If you want to suggest trying something new but aren't sure how your partner will feel, making it part of the fantasy is a good testing ground. Take a tie-up game. If he likes the idea (*She grabbed her discarded stockings and quickly bound him to the bed*) he'll continue the theme (*She tightened the knots around his wrists, sat back and gave a wicked grin. 'Now you're totally in my power'.*) If he doesn't, you'll find he'll quickly move onto another scenario (*But he broke free. 'I can't bear not being able to touch you', he said.*) In other words, forget it.

11 a.m.

- Make a list of the ten favourite things your partner does to you. You can be a bit sneaky with this one and make it instructional. 'I love it when you reach up to play with my breasts when you're giving me oral sex', might refer to the one solitary time he did that, but he'll certainly get the hint to do it a lot more in the future.

Noon

- Nip out for a coffee and take a quick detour to buy some gourmet goodies you can eat with your fingers, along with a treat like chocolates. This isn't the day for M&S sandwiches.

1 p.m.

- Depending on where you work/your cash situation, either meet at home for lunch or hire a cheap or posh hotel –

both have their appeal. Even if you've got as little as thirty minutes, don't underestimate what a bout of quick, urgent sex and sharing sensual food can do for your relationship. Seeing each other at a time of day you usually don't, makes things feel unfamiliar (a good thing if you've been together a while). It feels naughty nipping off from work to have sex in your lunch hour and has an affair-type feel, minus the tummy-turning guilt.

2 p.m.

- Given your slightly dishevelled appearance, it's probably best to busy yourself for a bit until your boss stops glancing over suspiciously. The second she/he does, reach into your handbag/desk drawer and whip out the erotic calendar you bought on the way back. Scribble a selection of sexual treats on various dates when you plan to deliver and 'Hi, honey, I'm home' takes on a whole new flavour.

3 p.m.

- Testosterone peaks for both men and women at around 3 p.m., so if you didn't have a sexy hook-up at lunchtime and you work close by, sweetly offer to buy coffee for the office and turn it into a chance to briefly meet (I really am going to get you sacked aren't I)! A coffee shop will do, but a park is better. If there are lots of people about, sit innocently on a bench and talk dirty to each other, describing what you'd do to each other if no-one was around. The saucier and naughtier the better. It's kinkier if people can actually eavesdrop, but it's not such a great idea when one could be the girl who cheerfully waves to you from reception. Everyone tittering behind their hands and a group email detailing what you said could almost make you regret doing it. Almost.

4 p.m.

- Make a list of ten new things you'd like to try over the next three months, then write down what you need to do to turn them into reality. If you've written 'spanking', you might need to buy a whip or paddle or invest in a book on the topic. If you're going to try anal sex, you not only need lubricant, you need to educate yourself on how to do it safely (see pages 104–5). When you've finished the list, decide which you need to check with your partner first before instigating and which you can surprise them with.

5 p.m.

- Call or text your partner to tell them how much you adore being with them and how much happier you are with them in your life. The most effective foreplay appeals to both our emotive and sexual sides.

6 p.m.

- Once you're home, go online and buy an erotic book or sex toy. Shopping via the internet means you can check out everything that takes your fancy without worrying what people think (see pages 281–6 for inspiration).

7 p.m.

- Pour a glass of champagne each and climb into a bubble bath together. You're not going to be there for ages, just a stolen ten or fifteen minutes before you get ready to go out. The idea is to get into the habit of doing sensual things together as well as sexual.

8 p.m.

- Instead of going straight to a restaurant for dinner, divert to a bar or place you've never been before for a pre-dinner drink. New surroundings help keep our senses stimulated and give us something new to talk about. 'People watch' and talk about how much sexier and in love you both are compared to all those other couples.

9 p.m.

- Move on to a restaurant with long tablecloths for dinner. This is where a floaty dress/no-knicker ensemble comes into its own. He starts by innocently putting one hand on her thigh under the table, while she inches forward to make it possible for him to slide his hand up, so he's stimulating her with his fingers. Both continue to chat casually and no-one need ever know he's actually bringing her to orgasm under the table. Some people are so good at this they can have a conversation with the waiter without stopping. Others, like me, get all embarrassed and flustered and end up ordering nine-inch instead of 9oz steaks and asking for 'no orgasms' instead of 'no oil'.

> *Couples who hold hands suffer less from stress and pain, according to researchers. But it only works if you're in love. Holding a stranger's hand doesn't have the same effect.*

10 p.m.
- When you get home you should both be so aroused that further foreplay isn't necessary. Shut the door behind you, check the kids are safely in bed and the babysitter paid and dispensed with, then rip off your clothes like they're suddenly soaked in battery acid and have intercourse across a table/on the floor/against a wall. Make sure it's a position you haven't tried before or in a place you've never done it.

11 p.m.
- Think it's all over because she's nodded off? This doesn't necessarily mean sex is over. I'm kidding, right? Well, sexpert Dr Glenn Wilson isn't. He sees nothing wrong with having sex with your partner while she's asleep, with her permission of course. He says that during sleep her vagina opens widely and 'a careful partner can lick her vulva and even insert several fingers without waking her'. Some women sleep so soundly they can be penetrated from behind without waking up. According to Dr Wilson, lots of women like waking up to find this happening while

they're semi-conscious and since many couples have different body clocks or levels of tiredness, it can be a way of compromising. Other women, however, might wake up and scream, 'Rape!' so *huge* emphasis should be placed on getting permission first! It's an idea which is a little out there and this means communication is crucial.

Midnight
- Get into spoon position, murmur 'I love you' then pass out. If you haven't already.

THE GROWN-UP'S GUIDE TO KISSING

Few events feel more like they should be trumpeted by angels than the first time you kiss the person you've liked/loved/slobbered over for ages. All those accidental touches, sitting a little too close, gazing hypnotized into each others' eyes, texting 50 million times a day, calling 4,000 times, their image burned onto the back of your eyelids (and all the while pretending this is normal behaviour) – all these things give little jolts of pleasure. But if you want to talk about most significant moments, the first kiss is usually up there for most couples. Some sets of mouths meet in a seamless, seemingly perfect fit, both of you kissing each other mirror style: confirmation you really have found your matching book end. (You might vomit now at such sickly clichés, but believe me, at the time that's how you thought.) At other times you'll bump noses and clash teeth, lust and passion sacrificing any attempt at technique, so desperate are you to eat each other up.

An open-mouthed kiss is the first signal couples use to show they find each other physically attractive and consider each other as potential sex partners. It's a big deal. Imagine then your utter and absolute disappointment when, after all that tortured build up, your first kiss leaves you dreading not desperate to go back for more. 'I felt like I'd been licked to death by an over-sized puppy dog'. 'It was like I'd tried to snog an ironing board'. 'He kept sticking his tongue down my throat to the point where I wanted to throw up.' 'It felt *wrong*. I think it was the whole thin-lips/full-lips thing'. Hmmm. Not quite what you were hoping for, eh?

The good news is that in most situations even the most incompatible kissers manage to sort things out so it's bearable. Which is fine. Sort of. Like, who really wants to spend the rest of their life having kisses which are bearable? For those who want a little more, I've come up with The Grown-up's Guide to Kissing. How to make that first time a little less traumatic and how to turn a bad kisser into a great one.

First-time pucker ups with someone new:
- Lust conquers many things but bad breath isn't one of them. Brush regularly, floss, get your teeth cleaned at the dentist, use mouthwash, drink lots of water and don't forget to scrape your tongue clean as well – you can buy tongue scrapers at any good chemist.
- Be aware, but try not to panic, that as you're kissing, your partner will instantly imagine how well you're likely to do when your mouth is attached to other parts. While you shouldn't kiss their mouth exactly the same way you intend to kiss their penis or vagina (that really would be odd!) you do need to give a hint of your style. Supersoft, slow and sexy? Fierce, passionate and confident? Both are good, but mixing them up is even better. Not so good is uncertain, slobbery, sloppy. Decide which type of kiss you're planning to start with before you go there.
- Relax your jaw and don't tense your mouth. Keep your lips soft and tilt your head slightly to one side. If you're nervous, cup their face or touch their chin so they know the kiss is coming – less chance of teeth clashing, which is highly embarrassing as a teen with braces but unforgivable when you might chip a new £1,000 veneer.

- Regardless of whether you've opted for tender or lusty, controlled passion is better at the start. As a general rule, though not a hard and fast one, it's better to start off soft and slow and move into fiercer, more forceful kissing.

- Sticking your tongue in too soon is like grabbing someone's breast with one hand while shaking their hand hello with the other. The right time for tongues is when your kisses have become a little more urgent, or you've been kissing for a while and someone has to up the ante.

- Open your mouth a little wider and with the tip rather than whole length of your tongue, move it back and forth, playing with their tongue or around the inside of their lips. Don't go too far in. If they give you tongue back, it means the sexual temperature is rising. If you want to, you can insert a little more tongue then and see how that's received.

- They liked it and the kisses have definitely moved from dreamy to hard, fast and deep? Time to move on to other parts, like kissing necks, and perhaps to add something else to the kiss – hands wandering tentatively to touch breasts/nipples through clothes etc.

How to turn a bad kisser into a good one:

You're actually not going to like the answer to this one because the solution isn't sneaky (well, maybe a tiny bit) and it involves directly confronting the problem – something most people hate doing. Well, brace yourself: being able to talk honestly and openly about sex is essential if you want anything near a decent relationship, so you might as well bite the bullet and do it now. (This exercise, by the way, works for kissing but also works for perfecting any technique.)

- If you want your partner to kiss you differently, you need to show them as well as tell them. That's right, give a demonstration. Rather than make this seem like an I'm-a-great-kisser-but-you-need-a-lesson exercise (even if it is!) tell your partner you read about a way to make kissing better. Say you want to be the best kisser they've ever had so how about giving it a whirl?

- Tell your partner the article said for both of you to imagine what you consider to be the perfect kiss, then demonstrate it to each other. Since they may already think you kiss perfectly, it's a good idea for you to (handily) go first. You were the one who read the story, remember, so it makes sense.

- Tell them verbally what you want, put as clearly and specifically as possible: 'My idea of the perfect kiss is one where we both have our mouths apart but not too much. There's a little bit of tongue but it's really more about moving our lips than our tongues.' That gives them a hint of what you want, but you can see why a demonstration is necessary. When we're talking about touch/kiss/lick instructions, it's so much easier to demonstrate than put into words.

- Kiss them the way you envisage this perfect kiss to be. Again, actually showing someone what you want sexually beats the hell out of even the most eloquent essay. Your partner shouldn't kiss back but remain as passive as possible, keeping their mouth soft and slightly open.

- Ask your partner what they thought. Did they understand what you want? Get them to repeat back key points then kiss you the way they think you'd like them to.

- Give them feedback and be positive but thorough. There's no point pretending they got it right if they didn't. It might take up to five trial kisses before they really get the hang of it.

- Repeat the exercise with both of you swapping roles.

- It depends on your partner's personality and how much they value your sexual satisfaction, but don't be surprised if all this gets forgotten the next time you kiss. You could take it as a personal insult when this happens, assuming they don't really care about pleasing you. Or you could assume they feel a little awkward and silly putting it all into practice. Give them the benefit of the doubt and remind them by saying, 'Hey, remember that kissing game we played? I loved the way you kissed me then. Can we do it that way?' Sometimes, though, it's not forgetting or not caring which makes them loath to show how much they learned the last time, it's resentment at you daring to instruct them. They were fine during the lesson but started stressing afterwards, when they'd had time to think about it, feeling they'd been unduly criticized. A good, honest chat should clear the air. If it doesn't, you've got two choices: leave or put up with a lifetime of sex on their terms. (Shall I call the cab or will you?)

THE SIX SECRETS TO GIVING A HELLISH HANDJOB

It's ironic, but most women I know are much more nervous about stimulating a man with their hands than they are about giving oral sex. The reason why women think they're phallus fumblers is mainly lack of practice. During those formative years, we'd give the odd squeeze through his jeans before things hotted up but once they did, he'd usually be the one doing it to us rather than vice versa. As a teenager, it's all about him getting us excited enough to go 'all the way', or putting our mouth where our hand is. Oral sex rather rapidly becomes the obvious favourite once you're actually 'doing it', and the humble hand-job takes second

> 'Don't be scared to grip the bloody thing! Penises are made of tough stuff and if you don't believe me, get him to masturbate for you. My girlfriend's first reaction was, "Jesus! Doesn't that hurt?"'
>
> James, 28

place. That's why I've gone back to basics with this step-by-step guide:

1. Pick your position: Are you left- or right-handed? Which is your best side? All too often, women try to deliver the goods in a position that feels uncomfortable or unnatural. You are allowed to *move*, you know! There's no need to make a big deal about it, simply roll over on top of him or straddle his lap, plant a long, slow, delicious kiss, then climb off onto the side that suits you. Don't be scared to deviate from the usual side-by-side position, either. Try him standing in front of you and you sitting on the edge of a bed, or him hovering above you, straddling your tummy as you lie on your back.

2. Use slippery stuff: When men do their own five-finger salute, they often slap on lubrication (if he doesn't, he has no idea what he's missing!). A dry penis is a sensitive one – it likes gentle stroking. Sliding your hand up and down (the standard male masturbation technique) can feel more like a vicious yank than an erotic you-know-what. Saliva is better than nothing, but clever girls come prepared with a tube of good-quality personal lubricant. He's used to using lube, so don't feel remotely embarrassed about squeezing some into your palm. Not *too* much though: being too generous is almost as bad as using none because it removes the friction entirely.

3. Get a grip: Sexperts worldwide dispense the same advice on this one: if you're a guy, touch her softer and slower, if you're a girl, touch him harder and faster. Lots of women make the mistake of being scared of his most prized part. Holding it between a finger and thumb, as though it's as fragile as spun glass isn't sexy, it just makes him think you don't want to touch it (not to mention giving him a complex about penis size. We all know the masturbation jokes where a tiny penis requires a finger and thumb, while Mr Massive gets a fist). Be nice, be firm and take a good, hard, confident hold, then move into a well-practised, confidently executed technique. Place all your fingers on one side, thumb on the other or make a loose fist.

4. Practise till you're a pro: If you read up too much about hand-job techniques you're liable to give up before you've even started. The instructions read like you're expected to reinvent the Rubik's cube. Try them out in practise, however, and you soon realize it's more like joining the dots. If you're keen to impress but don't want to look like an amateur in front of your new lover, practise on some props. A strategically positioned curtain rod, a carrot gripped between your thighs – virtually any cylindrical object will do. Yes, you'll feel like a right twit while you're doing it, but assuming you're not going to practise while watching your favourite soap with your flatmates, who cares? The basic motion you need to master is: slide up, circle and slide down the other side. Here's how it works: Grasp your hand firmly around the base of the penis and slide it upwards until it reaches the head.

In a study of 1,000 Norwegian men, it was the fifty-pluses who were enjoying sex the most. They were more sexually satisfied than men in their forties, and a lot happier than the least satisfied group: men in their thirties.

Once there, pause, rubbing the palm over the head in a small, sexy circle, then let your hand drop naturally down the other side of the penis, grasping the shaft until you're back at base camp again, but on the opposite side with your hand facing the opposite way. Try alternating, doing the same motion ten times with each lasting three to four seconds, then add one quick, firm pump-up-and-down stroke. Keep it going, adding an extra up-and-down pump each time. Make sure you decrease the number of pumps if he's dangerously close to losing it and you've got other plans for how to use that erection!

5. Employ back-up: Just use your hands and you risk having to dispense the longest hand-job in the entire world because of over-stimulation. No matter how deft and clever your handiwork, most men enjoy and often need extra stimulation to intensify and speed up the process of orgasm. So while one hand is working on his penis, use the other to cradle his testicles or stroke a nipple. Use your tongue on his testicles, nibble his neck, the inside of his thighs, his nipples. Try holding one hand in an 'L' position at the base of his penis, holding it firm as you work on him with your other hand. Not only does it make him look bigger – always a plus, even if he's the size of a fireman's hose – it creates heightened sensitivity. Putting pressure on the perineum just when you feel he's about to orgasm is especially effective.

6. Use props: If he, and you, are adventurous types – and if you aren't, why not? – use a small, cylindrical vibrator (called a wand vibrator) as well as your hands. Hold it on his testicles, perineum or use it to play around the opening of the anus. Alternatively, grab a silk scarf or strand of beads (check there aren't any rough edges first) wrap it around your hand or the shaft of his penis and slide it up and down the shaft and over the head.

🅕 FOR HER

Give him the finger

Inserting a finger into your partner's rectum during a hand-job, usually just before orgasm, will either make him love you forever or decide you're pure evil and never call you again. How to find out his reaction? Ask him if he'd like to try it, or start playing around the rim (the outside) of his anus and see what his reaction is. If he's nervous, it could be that he's concerned it will make him gay. The truth is, he's about as likely to turn gay from having a finger up there as I am to turn lesbian simply by wearing dungarees (many gay men, by the way, don't ever have anal sex). There's a great incentive for both of you to get over those ridiculous homophobic fears, though, because he could be in for the orgasm of his life. Like the clitoris, the root of the penis extends a few inches into his body. Stimulating the perineum massages the inner bit, but the true pleasure spot lies about three inches in. This is the prostate gland, nicknamed the male G-spot. To find it, and map its position for future reference, get him to lie on his back as you gently (and after using lots of lubrication) insert your index finger (palm up) almost all the way in. Aim towards his navel, then curve your finger in a 'come here' gesture.

Ⓜ FOR HIM

STICKY FINGERS
Techniques for touching her

Searching for that magic stroke that will reliably send her over the edge every time? Well you won't find it here. Sorry, lads, but such a stroke doesn't exist. Women are complex creatures and that's before we even talk about their even more complicated sexual systems. Depending on the time of the month, the mood we're in, whether we're having a fat day, have had too much to drink (or too little) or the cat's coughing up a fur ball . . . there are so many things that influence how we like to be touched at any particular time that you'd have to be bonkers to even attempt to understand it all. Besides, even if there was a wonder stroke, the body and mind tires of repetition and craves novelty. Which is why the following is only a guide to a simple, standard technique, which is a good starting point for most women. It's up to you to add your own flourishes (or you can cheat and buy *Hot Sex*, my first book, which includes all sorts of fancy finger dances)!

• If you're deadly serious about it and want to bring her to orgasm this way, use lubricant unless she's *very* wet. Place some on your fingers and apply it in one gentle, smooth stroke, starting from her anus and slowly drawing your fingers along her outer lips, before gently parting them and spreading the lubricant between her inner lips.

- Slide your middle finger gently between her inner lips, rocking it slightly from side to side as you do so. If you're doing it right, you'll feel her clitoris is engorged and standing to attention. Penises aren't the only things to get erections, you know!

- Let your finger come to rest on the clitoris and begin to make circles around the edges of it. Also try an up-and-down or diagonal movement. Keep your strokes light, consistent and continuous and be alert to her body language. If she lifts herself towards your hand, she probably wants a firmer touch. If she's pulling back slightly, go lighter. Listen for moans (good), altered breathing (good), if she goes suddenly quiet and tenses (very good – she could well be orgasming).

- Once she starts to move or thrust against you with her hips, insert one or two fingers deep inside her and make like a pretend penis. Alternate between the two techniques or position yourself so you can use two hands.

- Think about the angle of your finger as well as the movement. Most women like a nearly flat finger so you're using more of the pad than the tip. The pad is softer and you'll cover a greater area.

- Vary the sensation by using several fingers to slide between her inner lips, rather than just your middle one.

- There are two ways to stimulate her: by stroking the surface of the skin or by pressing and applying pressure. As a general rule, keep it even, smooth and constant when stroking and use rhythmic or continuous pressing when applying pressure.

- 'Peaking' is a technique which involves deliberately reducing or pausing stimulation so her level of arousal waxes and wanes. If it's early days and you're still learning her sexual triggers and how to read her body language, don't attempt it. Peaking is for couples who know exactly where their partners are on the orgasm cycle. If your partner's hovering around eight on a scale of one to ten stop directly stimulating her clitoris and move your hand up to massage her breasts and squeeze her nipples while kissing her. This might maintain her arousal level or cause it to drop. The trick is knowing when to recommence so it doesn't drop so low that the game stops being fun, or leaving it so late that it's all over. Stop stimulation as she's starting an orgasm at your peril (see page 77). Not good.

> 'I tried anal sex but my boyfriend was too big and it hurt. We've compromised by him using a small wand vibrator and inserting that instead. He gets turned on by doing it and it feels pleasurable for me as well. I think if you offer most men an alternative they aren't too upset about you saying no.'
>
> Debbie, 23

Ⓜ FOR HIM

Being anal about anal

Listen, I know 30–40 per cent of you have already tried anal sex, so this isn't meant to be a first-timer's guide. It's more of a gentle reminder of how to do it safely so *both* of you get pleasure (emphasis on the word gentle, right guys?)

- **Protect yourselves:** Faeces carry bacteria and anal play can spread HIV, hepatitis (A, B and possibly C), herpes, gonorrhoea, chlamydia and genital warts. Use condoms and don't ever put anything that's been in the anus straight into the vagina without thoroughly washing first. This goes for toys, too.

- **Don't even think about it if you don't have any lubricant:** If possible, use lubricant designed for anal sex, which is silicon- rather than water-based.
- **Stick a finger up your own bottom:** Yes, really. It's the only way you'll really understand how to make it as pain-free as possible. If you insert your finger about half an inch into your anus and press your fingertip against the side, you'll feel two sphincter muscles about a quarter of an inch apart. The 'outside' sphincter we have control over, the 'inside' sphincter is controlled by our autonomic nervous system, which basically means it does what it wants, when it wants, and it doesn't particularly like strange, unwanted things coming anywhere near it. If she says it's hurting, it's usually because this muscle has tensed around your penis, and the only way to stop this happening is to desensitize it. She can help enormously by inserting a finger inside herself every day for a few weeks. You can help by doing the same during sex and using sex toys designed for anal penetration. Bottoms are used to things coming out of them, not going in, so you need to build up to anal sex.
- **Be bloody careful:** When the muscles go into spasm, wait. If you don't wait for them to relax before continuing, it's not just going to hurt, it's going to *hurt like hell*! Anal sex is usually uncomfortable initially {some might say 'uncomfortable' is an understatement) but if she can relax, the pain recedes and pleasure replaces it.
- **Take it s–l–o–w:** Apply loads of lube and insert one or two fingers before introducing your penis. Then place the head against the opening and penetrate the head *only*. Insert a little at a time, checking with her at each stage. Once you're all in – and don't expect to fully penetrate on the

first try – stop and wait for her to relax around you. Get her to bear down, as though she's going to the toilet, which opens her anus.

- **Gentle thrusting, thanks:** While she may love a rigorous rodgering during vaginal intercourse, thrusting too fast or too deep while inside her bottom is not advised. Think slow and gentle.

4 Now *That* Hit The Spot!

How to orbit *your* orgasms

• •

At the risk of stating the obvious, sex is a fascinating topic for most of us. That's why sex 'sells' – it's the one thing that is never going to go out of fashion. Every time an apathetic forty-five-year-old decides sex is a bit boring and over-rated, there's a seventeen-year-old who's just discovered it and would trade five widescreen tellies for one glorious lick you-know-where from the yummy mummy next door. Massive amounts of money are being spent on sex, and I'm not talking about sex workers. Whether it's manufacturing a cutting-edge sex-toy range, researching the latest wonder drug or funding ground-breaking research, sex is the flavour of the millennium.

Volunteers have been filmed, prodded, interviewed, tape recorded, wired, monitored and measured for everything from their jumping blood pressure and contorted faces to their shallow gasps and arched backs and feet. But it's not just for the scientists' entertainment (come on, what would *you* rather study – a human having an orgasm or a rat trudging wearily round a treadmill?). The more we know about our arousal systems and why and how they work, the better able we are to understand and fix problems.

Not surprisingly, most of the research tends to focus on women. This isn't favouritism, it's because we're the ones who tend to have more complex sexual problems. The male arousal system is quite straightforward, whereas the female sexual system is complicated – and that's being kind. Orgasms for us can be more elusive than a single, attractive man aged thirty-five. Let alone one with even half his hair.

Feeling sad or stressed? Pucker up to your partner, but not during sex. According to US research, couples who kiss a lot in non-sexual situations are less likely to suffer from anxiety or depression.

For instance, it really would help to know why women orgasm at all. What evolutionary function does the female orgasm have? His is obvious: the more he sows his seed, the higher the chance of getting someone pregnant and keeping the world nicely populated – if a little overcrowded since Mother Nature possibly didn't appreciate how popular this activity would prove to be! Over the years, various theorists have had a stab at explaining why females climax. We have a clitoris, after all, and since it's designed purely for pleasure, it's obviously *supposed* to happen.

The Victorians considered the female orgasm both the cause and cure for hysteria – *Ha!* It did have a pay-off, though, since it led to the vibrator being invented and God knows where we'd be without that little device! Although hysteria – basically any malady which couldn't be explained by anything else – was exposed as a load of bollocks by the American Psychiatric Association in 1952, medical experts from the time of Hippocrates up to the twentieth century honestly believed it was the result of the womb being sexually deprived, and the standard cure was genital massage by your doctor. Yes, back in those days your local GP would manually masturbate you with the objective of inducing 'hysterical paroxysm' – otherwise known as an orgasm. Rather predictably, word spread fast and doctors couldn't keep up with the demand of women wanting to be 'cured' (i.e. get a sneaky hand-job) and so needed a way to get the job done faster. Enter the vibrator.

Darwinians figured that an orgasm kept a woman lying down after sex, handily keeping the sperm inside for longer and increasing her chance of conceiving. A theory clearly conceived by men used to being hit hard with the 'sleepy hormone', a chemical released into the male bloodstream a few minutes after orgasm and twenty minutes later in the female. Women can get a lot done in twenty minutes, so bang goes that theory! Others suggested orgasm evolved to bond couples, inspiring feelings of intimacy and trust (sweet); another experiment showed the cervix dips during orgasmic contractions, helping to give the semen underneath it a leg-up on its mission to meet an egg (sensible).

The most recent theory is perhaps the most ambitious, suggesting orgasm is a sophisticated means of women subconsciously choosing which of her lovers she wants to father her children. Researchers asked volunteers to keep track of the timing of their orgasms during sex and to collect his ejaculate from vaginal 'flowback' – the stuff which comes back out again, usually several hours later, just when you're sitting down at his parents' for Sunday lunch. Three hundred sessions and sperm samples later, they found that when a woman climaxes any time between a minute before to forty-five minutes after her lover ejaculates, she retains significantly more sperm than she does after sex that doesn't include an orgasm.

Armed with this nugget of information, they coupled it with another. Several studies show symmetrical people are not only seen as more attractive, they're physically and psychologically healthier than the less symmetrical. So it follows that if women's orgasms are an adaptation for securing good genes for offspring, women should report more orgasms with symmetrical partners. And guess what? They do. Put it all together and you come up with this: an orgasm means women retain sperm for longer, upping the chances of conception, and they have more orgasms with the genetic favourite, Mr Symmetrical. So the likelihood of conceiving these men's children is significantly higher. The moral of the story: if you sleep with a particularly attractive man, for God's sake use contraception.

Another significant advance: female orgasm appears to be more about letting go than getting all hot and bothered. Gert Holstege, who spoke at a sex therapy conference I attended recently, had the rather brilliant idea of using an MRI machine to measure brain activity during orgasm. Well, it seems like a brilliant idea until you consider the logistics: a) finding a hospital that will allow people to orgasm inside one and b) figuring out how the hell to give someone an orgasm while inside, given that they're a long tunnel designed to house just one (usually very nervous rather than very horny) person, with no real room to DIY. Happily, Gert had solutions. He persuaded a hospital to let him use their machine on Saturdays and got volunteer couples to take turns lying inside the machine while their partner reached in from the outside and brought them to orgasm by hand. Bizarre? Yes! But even more so when I found out that the person masturbating their partner had to give exactly eight minutes warning of when they would climax because of the way the MRI machine measures activity. Enlightening? Incredibly. What Gert uncovered however, was initially alarming.

Pictures of the male brain showed that parts of it light up like a Christmas tree during orgasm, while the same picture of the female brain showed . . . nothing. Bugger all. Hardly even a flicker. Nearly every female in the audience shifted uncomfortably at this news, and looked a little perplexed. We'd all had orgasms (at least I assume so; it would be a slight worry if a sex therapist hadn't managed it) and it felt like fireworks to us, so why wasn't it activating our brain cells? Gert then had a brain wave, literally: if the cells weren't activating, maybe they were doing something else? So he measured *de*activation during orgasm and surprise, surprise, there was a result. This time it was the female brain that lit up, while the males' didn't.

It turns out that the part of the brain that governs emotional control – things like fear and anxiety – switch off when a woman is having an orgasm. Orgasm for us is about letting go – stopping feeling and thinking, and not letting stress get in the way. Deactivation of these important parts of the brain might be the most important necessity for women having an orgasm.

So what do you know? It's taking an awfully long time but we are gradually piecing together a detailed picture of just what the hell is going on down there, not to mention every-where else. In this chapter, I've used the latest research as a base for devising some practical applications to make your orgasm experience a more enjoyable one.

ARE ORGASMS PRE-PROGRAMMED FROM BIRTH?

Here's something else you can blame Mum and Dad for: your sex drive. Two significant gene studies have thrown up some rather interesting results. First up, around 30 per cent of people appear to carry a heightened arousal gene mutation which gives them an erotic edge on the rest of us. Less lucky are the people who carry another gene which dampens arousal and sex drive.

Another study found a woman's ability to have an orgasm is at least in part determined by her genes. ➤

A London research team studied 4,037 female twins – half identical, half non-identical – and found a definite genetic influence on the ability to reach orgasm. They found that genes are responsible for why 34 per cent of the women couldn't climax through intercourse and 45 per cent of them couldn't orgasm during masturbation. Which is a sort of good-news, bad-news scenario. On the one hand, it's pointless feeling guilty if you can't climax because it's not in your control. On the other, it's desperately disheartening to think you're pre-programmed not to enjoy sex as much as other women. Conscious of this, the researchers stress the 'unfortunate' gene packages don't mean you're doomed, just that you and your lover need to invest a little more time and effort into lovemaking. Sorted.

COME TOGETHER

I'm writing this section a little bit under duress. I *so* don't want to perpetuate the myth that a) there's something wrong with one or both of you if you don't have simultaneous orgasms as often as you clean your teeth, or b) it's the be-all and end-all orgasm experience. Quite frankly, taking turns is not only more practical – it's much harder to come together than it is in succession – it's sometimes a lot more satisfying. Having an orgasm is a selfish experience: you're totally and utterly fixated on your own pleasure, which means it's bloody difficult to pay much attention to your partner's. For men, this is less of a problem. Their orgasms are easier to trigger and once triggered they continue. Women's require a lot more attention and, unless tended from start to finish, can halt halfway through. While he's twitching and moaning with orgasmic joy, she's often twitching and moaning with resentment at having been robbed at the last moment. Yes it can be an incredibly bonding moment when it does all come together – ahem – but you're still better off making it a pleasant bonus rather than an aim. I also want to reiterate, even if you are mighty sick of hearing me say it, that most women *don't* orgasm purely through penetration. So if you're feeling inferior about not having coital orgasms, stop being silly. You're the norm, not the sad exception.

This guide is about how to orgasm together through penetration, but don't ignore other ways, like masturbating together or having a 'sixty-niner'. I'm also generalizing in order to appeal to as many of you as possible. Most of the time, spontaneous orgasm is about getting him to slow down (i.e. not orgasm so quickly) and getting her to speed up (hurry up hers). If the opposite is true for you, some of the tips won't apply. If this is you, read the ones for the opposite sex and you may find they're more applicable.

> 'I spent most of my life faking orgasms whenever my partner had one because I thought they wouldn't want to be with me if I didn't. Then one day I just got fed up. I told my husband of two years that I'd been faking and was only able to have an orgasm through oral sex; he smiled and said, "I thought so". Men aren't as stupid as you think.'
>
> Megan, 41

Ⓜ FOR HIM

- **Have an orgasm first:** and make the 'together' orgasm the second one. Most men find they have much better control second time around.
- **Stop thinking about the orgasm:** you're about to have and instead focus on how fabulous the sensation you're feeling now is. Forget old advice about doing the opposite and trying to distract yourself completely. Tasks like counting backward from 500 are marginally useful

(and I've been guilty of suggesting it myself) but new research shows that even as you're manically saying '346' in your brain, another part is saying 'What does he think I am, stupid? As if this is going to grab my attention when I've got a pair of breasts bobbing in front of me, my penis is nestled in a nice, warm, sexy place, my girlfriend's moaning and throwing her head back and . . . Right, now that's over with, we really can concentrate – 345, 344 . . .' It's the old pink elephant syndrome – tell yourself not to think of pink elephants and that's all your brain will conjure up.

It seems the trick isn't to remove yourself from the situation but to stay very much in the moment. Sure you're waiting until she's ready, but this doesn't mean you have to sexually twiddle your thumbs. Women aren't the only ones who can hover in the plateau stage: totally turned on but not out of control. The better you can do this, the keener you are to take your time during sex – and the higher the chances of her being satisfied and the two of you reaching that glorious climax together. Achieve this by trying the next technique.

- **Know your orgasm inside out:** so you know exactly what's going to send you over the edge. The easiest way to do this is to get into the habit of 'scoring' where you're at. Think about your last great orgasm moment and that gets a ten. Zero is when you're at your in-laws making small talk in between passing the brussel sprouts, i.e. no arousal at all. As you move from no arousal to lift-off, you'll move through the spectrum from one to ten. Practise rating yourself and you'll have much more control over when you orgasm, i.e. 'I'm hovering around the six mark, so I can afford to keep thrusting hard for a bit longer' or 'I'm definitely an eight, so I'd better stop or switch stimulation until I calm down'. Lots of men find it easier to practise assessing their arousal levels during masturbation so they can focus exclusively on the task. After you think you've got it mastered, work out what your average degree of arousal is in sex. Think back to your last four sex sessions and grade them on how you felt the majority of the time. You're doing well if arousal hovers around seven or eight for an average session: you're getting a lot of enjoyment but you're relatively in control.

- **Stop or switch stimulation if you climb higher than an 'eight':** If you're having intercourse, stop moving and relax inside her for a minute or so. If she's giving you oral sex, get her to come up for air and give you a nice long snog. Or simply stop and do absolutely nothing. If you're giving her oral sex and it's turning you on so much you think you're closer to orgasm than she is, do the same – and maybe give pages 77–82 a quick read to check on your technique while you're at it!
- **Make friends with her vibrator:** If you asked me the best tip I could possibly give you to achieve simultaneous orgasm, this would be it. One of you holding a wand vibrator – slim, cylindrical, non-intrusive – over the clitoral area during penetrative sex is (in my opinion anyway) the most effective way to ensure a shared orgasm experience. Why don't more people do it? Some don't like introducing something 'mechanical', and lots of men don't understand the whole vibrator thing and feel a tad threatened – yes, even you! Quite frankly, in terms of fast, guaranteed, regular orgasms there *is* no competition. Women have problems *not* having an orgasm with a vibrator, rather than *having* one. Having said this, you still shouldn't be threatened. Jealous, yes, but not threatened. It's not like they're human. The closest you can get to becoming a human vibrator is to

attach a tiny vibrator to your tongue or penis. Happily, both devices are available and actually work very well (see pages 281–3).

On other occasions, such as trying for simultaneous orgasms during intercourse, you really do need to accept defeat, reach into the bedside table drawer and pull it out (that's the vibrator, not you).

🅕 FOR HER

- **Tease yourself during masturbation:** Use the same technique as he does (see pages 114–5) to find out how you rate at any given moment. Few women climb steadily from one to ten, spending the same amount of time at each level. Most skip all over the place in an average sex session, going from a three to a six if he hits the right spot with his tongue and sliding from nine to three if he doesn't. The trick for simultaneous orgasm is to get you as close as possible to tipping over, but leaving enough time for him to catch up. Luckily for both of you, it's usually a matter of seconds, let alone minutes.

- **Use lubrication** and make sure he understands it doesn't mean you're not turned on if you're not wet. It's a good indicator but it's not absolute and it's also individual: some women lubricate loads, others only a tiny amount when they're so horny they'd trade the three kids for three flicks of the right tongue.

- **Use the bridge technique:** This is the manoeuvre most sex therapists recommend. The basic idea is to give you clitoral stimulation up to the point of, but not actually to, orgasm and let his thrusting trigger off the orgasmic reflex. This effectively provides a 'bridge' between clitoral stimulation and intercourse. He stimulates the clitoris right up to penetration, then thrusting takes over as the prime stimulation. Some studies show that up to half of women who couldn't previously climax through penetration alone were able to, without priming first, after using this technique regularly.

- **Choose the right position:** Woman on top or him from behind are the most likely positions to stimulate the front vaginal wall and up your chances of orgasm. Some men say her-on-top makes it easier for them to control ejaculation; others say that being so visual and having that glorious view has the opposite effect. Decide which positions are most likely to tip you over the edge and pray like hell it's one that has the opposite effect on him.

- **Pull out all the stops:** Try all the techniques solo and if they don't work (or even if they do) combine them. Pick a position that hits the front wall of the vagina *and* use a wand vibrator on your clitoris. One of you works on your clitoris as he penetrates *and* bites your neck, talks dirty or does whatever your personal orgasm trigger might be.

- **Use your PC muscle to control orgasms:** The better toned your genitals, the more control you'll have over both your orgasms. Not only can you 'milk' him with your muscles when you're ready for him to orgasm, pretty much ensuring he will too, rhythmically squeezing your PC muscle is thought to increase lubrication and your pleasure as well.

- **If you think he's too close to climaxing:** and you're not ready yet, pull down on his testicles gently to decrease his chances of orgasm. Keep your hands *away* from his perineum, testicles or anus until you're ready for him to climax. Double stimulation for him isn't usually a good idea until you're almost 100 per cent there.

- **Talk lots:** telling each other exactly where you're at. I don't mean a clinical, doctor-like discussion – 'I'm at 4.678 moving steadily toward a 5. But hang on, that's just dipped to 4.4544' – more along the 'God this is great! I'm nearly there, honey' lines. If you don't think it will interfere with the mood, use the number system. Groaning out a 'Nine!' or delivering a curt '*Still* two,' might seem odd to start, but it's a quick and effective way to communicate in bed.

- **Masturbate in front of each other:** taking turns, and concentrating on watching your partner's body signs at each stage. This will give you lots of clues as to how excited your partner is at any given moment.

- **Let your arousal levels dictate what to do next:** He's a six and she's a nine? This is the moment to move into fast, furious penetrative sex with the best chance of both of you coming together through penetration. He's a nine and she's a six? Cease his stimulation entirely and get him to concentrate on her with his fingers, mouth, a vibrator . . .

- **Switch stimulation regularly:** Not only will it keep you both hovering rather than climbing steadily towards a climax, it stops sex becoming too orgasm-focused. Change positions. Massage, lick or caress each other's nipples. Give oral sex, receive it, change rooms, change the CD – anything to alter the mood, keeping it hot and sexy but maintaining a measure of control.

REPEAT AFTER ME . . .
Yes, I talk a lot about how to control your orgasms and make them better, bigger, deeper, wetter and wilder, but

while the underlying theme is always how to have the best sex you possibly can, ensure you don't lose sight of the big picture by adopting the following three rules as your orgasm mantra.

- **You don't give your partner an orgasm and they don't give you one:** Each person is responsible for reaching his or her own orgasm. Only you know what you need and want and it's up to you to communicate this to your partner.
- **The best way to maximize your orgasm is to minimize the importance of achieving one:** Sex should be about the journey not the destination.
- **No two orgasms feel the same and there are a lot of factors influencing them which really are out of your control:** Your general mood, how tired you are, the amount of time since your last orgasm, the time of the month, medication you're on – all of these have an effect. And that's without taking into account emotional factors like who's stimulating you (your lover of ten years or Jesse Metcalfe from *Desperate Housewives*), how you feel about them (bored/so excited you're practically hyperventilating), your expectations (low/high is the understatement of the century). Rather interestingly, scientists who've measured the intensity of muscle contractions find they don't necessarily correspond with how satisfying the orgasm felt. It might seem like you're blasting off the Richter scale, but it's your brain that's beating records, not your body.

COME AGAIN

If one orgasm is difficult for some, having two is tougher for just about all of us. Why? After you've 'taken the edge off' our nerve endings become desensitized, we're often emotionally satisfied and our bodies start flooding with hormones designed to make us believe once is enough. While you might want to make love all night long, your body probably doesn't. Researchers at a German university believe prolactin, the hormone linked to sperm and breast milk production, may flood the body after orgasm, signalling to the body that it's had enough. Measuring hormone levels in women who'd been asked to masturbate to orgasm (don't quit your day job, research subjects get paid a pittance) researchers discovered a surge in several hormones, but the rise of prolactin was the most dramatic and prolonged. Since prolactin regulates dopamine, the neurotransmitter which plays a role in governing pleasure and pain, it could be that this surge acts as a type of cut-out switch, signalling to the brain that it's time for beddy-byes rather than more action. Since both sexes release prolactin, it's believed that the same process also occurs in men.

Before we go any further with the whole concept of multiple orgasms, let's define them. First up, for him, we have the infamous non-ejaculatory orgasm – think Sting rather than an enthusiastic eighteen-year-old, able to perform three times in one session with a mere ten minutes between orgasms. The NEO is when he experiences orgasm in his brain but inhibits ejaculation using his PC muscle and/or other techniques whilst retaining his erection. Another way of having multiple orgasms is via multiple-ejaculation – now think of the eighteen-year-old. He has several orgasms in a row, all accompanied by full or partial ejaculation. Some men lose their erection fully each time while others maintain it. In this case, it's usual for the first orgasm to be the most intense; masters of non-ejaculatory orgasms claim each and every climax is as intense as the last (show-offs!).

For women, a multiple can mean one, super-long, über-orgasm or lots of orgasms in one sex session. Because women don't fall to the post-orgasm resolution phase as quickly as a man does, it's easier for us to climb back up and have further orgasms in succession. The percentage of women who experience multiple orgasms has tripled from 14 to over 50 per cent since the fifties, compared to 12 per cent of the male population. But just as lots of couples don't bother trying to have simultaneous orgasms, multiple orgasms don't appeal to everyone either. For men, there's the laziness factor. Training yourself to be multi-orgasmic takes effort ('Why not just have one big one and go to sleep?' said a male friend of mine perplexed why anyone would go to all that trouble). And not everyone wants, or has time for the long, drawn-out sex session that's usually necessary to produce them. But even if you don't think multiples are your cup of tea, doing the following should result in better quality orgasms generally.

> **❶ Think you're pretty hot? Sexologist Beverly Whipple studied a man who experienced six orgasms in thirty-six minutes with no erection loss!**

Ⓜ FOR HIM

- **Use different stimulation for each orgasm:** If you're aiming for the ultimately easier option of having several orgasms with ejaculation per session, the trick is to have them via different means. If you have your first via intercourse, you've got more chance of having another through oral sex than through more penetrative sex. A third might be achievable through masturbating – it's going to be the hardest to have so call in the expert (you).
- **Take your time:** Men are no different to women when it comes to orgasm intensity: the longer the action, the stronger the reaction. There's good evidence that the

strength of your orgasm, like hers, depends on the length of foreplay and other erotic stimulation involved. While you can both masturbate to orgasm in a few minutes (you through masturbation, her with a vibrator) it feels more satisfying when you've hovered at the 'plateau' stage – the stage after arousal and before orgasm.

- **Know what you're aiming for:** This is the basic premise you need to absorb for non-ejaculatory orgasms: orgasm and ejaculation might go together like strawberries and cream, but they are in fact two separate processes. An orgasm is something you feel in your brain, an ejaculation is physical: your body pumping out semen through a series of contractions. As I said earlier, men who have multiple orgasms have mastered the ability of having an orgasm in their head, without ejaculating and losing their erection in the process. They might display all the usual outward signs of orgasm – twitching, groaning, that weird 'orgasm face' she's grown to love – but their penis stays hard and they're able to go again, and sometimes again and again. How do they do it? Here's the bad news: it's bloody difficult and requires time, effort, discipline and bucket-loads of motivation. Why bother? Quite apart from impressing the hell out of her, multi-orgasmic men say if you train yourself well, orgasms can be felt through the entire body rather than being penile centric. While the average bloke is usually completely and utterly knack-ered after a mere two ejaculations, a multi-orgasmic man feels energized, bounding into the kitchen to fix a nice beansprout and tofu salad, after six.
- **Get into training:** If you're deadly serious about this, I would strongly recommend investing in some good books on the topic and *The Multi-Orgasmic Man* by

Mantak Chia and Douglas Abrams Arava is an excellent start. The truly committed who also live in a major city will find there are weekend workshops and courses you can enroll in. Look up 'spiritual sex' on the web, flick through mags like *Time Out*, call up a reputable sex shop in your area and ask for recommendations. Be aware that a lot of these courses are rubbish (the 'expert' is someone more adept at fleecing you for cash than cranking your love life up a gear) and often attract people who think it's a cover for swinging (don't get too excited, intelligence isn't the only thing these people are lacking). Call up and ask for qualifications and what the workshops involve and you'll soon get an idea of how helpful it's likely to be. Chia and Arava recommend you Google 'Healing Tao instructor' to see if there's one in your area. They come highly recommended and teach classes and workshops in things like Sexual Kung Fu(!). A good workshop will focus on spiritual and mental exercises which teach you how to get full – or as close to full as possible – control over your body and bodily functions. You'll also do a lot of work on your PC muscle and discover the role it plays in inhibiting ejaculation. Something to note is that a side effect of curing premature ejaculation – learning ejaculation control – is sometimes spontaneous multiple orgasms! Like I said, though, you'd want to be committed.

A study of 20,000 sixteen- to twenty-four-year-olds in the UK found that nearly a third lost their virginity before they were sixteen and 4 per cent lost it before they were fourteen.

F FOR HER

- **Use different stimulation for each orgasm:** Just like him, you've got a better chance of having more than one orgasm if it's via a different means.
- **Breathe:** How you breathe is important. Some experts say holding your breath on orgasm heightens the sensation, others say if you starve your brain of oxygen, it forces oxygen-giving blood to flow towards it and *away* from your genitals. Continuing to breathe deeply through orgasm is recommended by spiritual sex devotees, who claim it means you're more likely to have a second one. While yet more experts say if you want to feel your orgasm over a wider area, start with regular deep breaths and then start panting just before orgasm. Who's right? It's about what works for you, so give them all a try.

> *Writing makes the heart grow fonder. Research at the University of Texas found that when at least one partner wrote his or her deepest feelings about the relationship, 77 per cent were still together three months later, compared to 52 per cent who wrote about everyday activities.*

- **Know what you're aiming for:** As much as most orgasms follow a similar pattern, they vary enough between individuals for some experts to claim we each have our very own 'orgasm fingerprint'. One theory about female orgasm says there are two distinct nerves responsible for the two different 'basic' orgasms, clitoral and front wall. The pudendal nerve goes to the clitoris and the pelvic nerve goes to the vagina and uterus. Because the pudendal has more nerve endings, this could be why women have more clitoral than vaginal orgasms. The two nerves actually overlap in the spinal cord, which may explain why women are able to have 'blended' orgasms – clitoral and front wall simultaneously. Several factors seem to influence whether women have both multiple and vaginal orgasms: the strength of their PC muscles, the sensitivity of their G-spots and other internal spots, motivation to keep trying different stimulation and orgasm triggers. As a general rule, the more ways you're able to orgasm, via masturbation, oral, front wall etc., the more likely you are to have multiple orgasms.

- **Get into training:** First up, do your 'Kegels'. The PC muscle supports the pelvic floor and spasms during orgasm. Like the rest of your body, if it's toned and fit it works better, pumping even more blood to the pelvis, which is great for arousal, and making stronger contractions which will give longer, more intense orgasms. Which means – and I apologize for this – that on top of those laborious gym sessions, made bearable only by those little tellies installed on the treadmill, you need to add Kegel workouts. Happily, these take minutes rather than hours and you can do them anywhere. Simply squeeze the muscle you use to hold back urine, hold it for two seconds, then release, and do this twenty times, three times per day.

- **Practise 'peaking' techniques:** As I explained on page 104, peaking involves taking yourself *almost* to the point of orgasm, waiting for your arousal to subside, then climbing back up again. This trains you to stay in a high state of excitement, following a wave-like orgasm pattern, rather than one which starts at the bottom and steadily climbs higher. Not only does this optimize the release of endorphins – hormones which naturally take us to a place we try to artificially induce with twenty-five glasses of wine and five tequila shots – it teaches your body to stay in a practically permanent orgasmic pleasure zone, able to orgasm over and over again.

- **Deliberately develop orgasm triggers:** The more your brain travels a certain path neurologically, the more effortless it becomes. Curving your lips upward lets your brain know you're happy, triggering the release of serotonin, a hormone which makes you feel happy as well as look it. The more signposts of impending orgasm your brain can recognize, the easier it will be to trigger the orgasmic response. Focus on what you naturally do on approach to orgasm, then exaggerate it. If you breathe heavier and faster, breathe even heavier the next time you're about to climax. If you notice you tense your toes and throw your head back, do that. Get to the point where your brain thinks, *Aha!* Deep heavy breathing combined with toe flexing means she's about to orgasm (better get cracking then and make it happen). Do this and orgasm becomes effortless and spontaneous. (Just don't get over-excited in meetings during a long leg stretch.)

> 'The first time is easy, the second time I need more stimulation. He puts three fingers inside me and curves them upward, then he puts his thumb on my clitoris and makes little circles with it.'
>
> Jade, 23

I'LL HAVE WHAT SHE'S HAVING...

One US study on multiple orgasms concentrated, rather sensibly, on 805 nurses – not only are they anatomically well-educated and know their own bodies better than most, they're less embarrassed about being questioned about sex. Comparing the nurses who had multiple

---

orgasms to those who didn't, the researchers found that women who have multiples:

- Discovered pleasure at an early age – they're the little girls who embarrassed the hell out of their mothers by 'riding' the arm of the sofa, rubbing themselves furiously while prudish Aunt Sally watched with amazement.
- Are more likely to have examined their own clitoris. They got the hand mirror out and had a good old look, usually during their teens.
- Enjoy giving and receiving oral sex.
- Like their breasts and nipples fondled, kissed and bitten.
- Straddle their partner's thigh or masturbate themselves to enhance clitoral stimulation during intercourse.
- Enjoy erotic fantasies, films and books, both solo and with a partner.
- Take an active role during sex. Their multiple orgasms don't happen by accident, they know what they need, know what techniques work best for them and, most crucially, tell their partners.
- Choose partners who are sensitive and sexually and emotionally intelligent (so they're clever all round obviously).
- Tend to form stable, satisfying relationships, possibly because they're able to satisfy their sexual needs effectively.

THE FAB FOUR
Hot zones for her

In case you haven't noticed, there's a lot of money being pumped into sex research these days. Kinsey-type research institutes are popping up all over the place and any number of startlingly intimate experiments are being conducted at this

> **The reason why two out of three women don't orgasm from penetration alone is because we use 'monotonous' intercourse positions, says zoologist Desmond Morris. When twenty-seven couples were asked to shake things up, using positions which accessed their G- and A-spots, three-quarters of the females reported regular vaginal orgasms.**

very moment. The result isn't just a wealth of new material for greedy little sexperts like me to pounce on, we now know so much more about how the body's arousal system works. And guess what? Turns out the clitoris, our good old faithful orgasm 'button', isn't the only spot guaranteed to make our knickers fizz. If the secret to having a maximum number of orgasms per session is switching stimulation to different erogenous zones, the more they discover the better, quite frankly. Fancy a night of unequalled orgasmic bliss? Get your partner to work his way through the alphabet in one session, stimulating each of these erotic centres in rotation.

Number one son: The Clitoris

What is it? Let's take a moment to raise our glasses to the humble clitoris: after all, it's the only organ in the human body whose purpose is purely pleasure. Men don't have one, only women do (tee hee) which goes a little way to making up for all the other stuff we have to suffer and they don't (periods, pregnancy, pointy shoes, PMT ... and that's just the Ps). When stimulated, the clitoris swells, lengthens and becomes more erect, making it even more sensitive. Most of the clitoris is hidden beneath the surface. Australian urologist Helen O'Connell studied cadavers and found that the part you see is, in fact, just the tip. It's attached to an inner mound of erectile tissue the size of your first thumb joint. That tissue then breaks into two 'legs' which extend another eleven centimetres *and* there are also two clitoral 'bulbs' which run down the area just outside the vaginal opening. All this tissue is erectile – it enlarges or swells with stimulation – and contributes to orgasmic muscle spasms. So it's really a lie to say some women can orgasm without clitoral stimulation because the act of thrusting alone massages the hidden parts of the clitoris. 'There will therefore always be some degree of clitoral stimulation, even when the tip is not touched directly,' says zoologist Desmond Morris.

How to find it: It's at the top of the vulva. If you put your finger on your vaginal opening, then draw it upward between your inner lips, you'll feel a little nub partially covered by a protective hood. This is the visible part of the clitoris. Just like his penis, the size of the clitoris differs between individuals. It could be the size of an erect nipple or way bigger.

The likelihood of you having an orgasm this way: With so much tissue involved, it's no wonder clitoral orgasms are the easiest to have. Just the tip of the clitoris has 7–8,000 nerve fibres. Women find it easier to climax from oral, digital or mechnical stimulation of the clitoris than any other way.

Roadtest: 'I'm one of those lucky women who can also climax through penetration but clitoral orgasms, without a shadow of a doubt, are far more intense. If I had to choose between the two, they win by a long shot.' *Jenny, 35*

New kid on the block: The U-spot

What is it? If parts of our bodies were bars and restaurants, this spot would currently be the coolest, hippest place in town. American researchers recently unveiled the erotic potential of the U-spot by discovering women had a powerful sexual response when the area was gently stimulated by a finger, tongue or tip of the penis. The urethra is being implicated sexually in a lot of experiments. During research into

Femidom, the rather embarrassing, unsuccessful, female condom, ultrasound imaging confirmed that the front wall of the vagina and urethra are stretched significantly during intercourse. It's suspected the stretching causes the urethra to release 'happy hormones' like serotonin from cells in the urethral wall, so it also plays a part in the arousal process.

How to find it: Look for a small patch of sensitive erectile tissue just above and on either side of the urethral opening. The urethra is the tiny hole pee comes out of and it's usually midway between your vaginal opening and clitoris. Get him to concentrate on this area with his tongue or finger (use lubrication unless you're really wet). During intercourse, spread your legs wide, pressing yourself against his penis and pelvis to allow maximum contact, and get him to grind rather than thrust.

Likelihood of you having an orgasm this way: It's a bit like the G-spot: some women swear it's scream material, others don't get it at all. But it's easy to pinpoint and experiment with, so give it a whirl and keep up the stimulation for a good five minutes before dismissing it entirely as just another fad.

Roadtest: 'Not only did I orgasm, it felt completely different to my usual clitoral orgasm. It was easy to find and I'm now a huge fan.' *Toni, 25*

The old favourite: The G-spot or front wall

What is it? If you've never heard of the G-spot, you really should get out more. Such a small thing, such controversy. When researchers first discovered this area was sexually sensitive, women's magazines and the media went berserk. Assuming they'd found a 'sex button' that guaranteed fast, furious, universe-moving orgasms on demand, the whole country stayed inside for a week, poking and prodding about trying to find theirs. Most failed – mainly because such a button doesn't exist (dammit). Some still maintain the G-spot is nothing but a decadently optimistic fantasy but others say there does appear to be a small, sexually responsive patch on the vaginal wall which can trigger orgasm when stimulated, which would explain why G-spot dildos or vibrator attachments are becoming more and more popular. I'm sticking with my initial theory: while there are areas on the front vaginal wall that are sensitive when stimulated, the exact location of these hotspots varies from individual to individual.

How to find it: Personally, I think you're better off stimulating the whole of the front vaginal wall and going with the spot that feels good to you. The front vaginal wall, by the way, is the side closest to your tummy. The classic 'G-move' is for him to insert and curve his fingers, making a 'come here' motion, or to get into a position where his penis has a direct target, with him behind or you on top. If you're looking for the specific location of the G-spot, it's supposedly 5–8 cm (2–3 inches) inside the vagina on the front or upper wall. The area protrudes slightly, but only when the glands surrounding the urethral tube have become swollen. In other words, you're not likely to find it if you start having a poke around while loading dishes in the dishwasher, but you may if you're in the process of having fantastic sex with the hot, young man sent to install it.

Likelihood of you having an orgasm this way: If we're talking general front-wall stimulation, the chances of you climaxing are good. If you're determinedly setting off on a G-spot expedition, grimly clutching a compass, you've probably

> *Married people are never happy with their sex lives, or are they? Despite the bad press, one study showed that 63 per cent of American men say their sex life is better now that they are married and 94 per cent say they are happier overall than when they were single.*

got a 40/60 chance. Some women apparently don't have one and others hate the sensation because it's too intense.

Roadtest: 'I was the biggest sceptic until I went out with a guy who used to search quite deliberately till he found a certain spot, then rub it with amazing results. He claimed it was the G-spot, I have no idea where it was because the second he hit it, I'd lose concentration.' *Sara, 31*

Last but sooo not least: The A-spot

What is it? The anterior fornix crogenous is a patch of sensitive tissue at the inner end of the vaginal tube between the cervix and the bladder. It's apparently the female equivalent of his prostate, and we all know that's the technical term for what is essentially the male G-spot. According to A-spot devotees, direct stimulation of this spot doesn't just produce orgasms, the contractions are so strong they're almost violent. Another bonus: unlike other spots such as the clitoris, the A-spot is reputed not to suffer from over-sensitivity after orgasm. Which, of course, means there's no need to stop at just one.

How to find it: Just like the G-spot, there's slight confusion over where the A-spot is. It was initially thought to be halfway between the 'G-spot' and the cervix, but the latest person to document it, zoologist Desmond Morris, says it's actually a patch of sensitive tissue just above the cervix, between it and the bladder, at the innermost point of the vagina. It's not clear whether Masters and Johnson (US sex researchers) are talking about the A-spot when they describe 'tenting', but it sounds a lot like it to me. They say that when a woman becomes really aroused, the muscles and ligaments surrounding the uterus lift it up and 'tent', allowing penetration into an extra inch or so of space behind the cervix. The result: incredible orgasmic sensations.

Likelihood of you having an orgasm this way: At the risk of giving too much information, this one rivals the clitoris for me.

The trouble is, the guy has to have ridiculously long fingers to reach it. My boyfriend at the time was 6ft 5inches, with fingers in proportion to his height, and by God did he know what to do with them. It's now possible to buy A-spot vibrators – long, thin and curved upward at the end (for those who don't have hands like ET's), long fingers and specially shaped vibrators tend to be a lot more effective than a penis. You'll know when you've hit it because it's like someone just opened the floodgates as it tends to produce rapid lubrication.

> 'I don't thrust, I move in circles. Then I'll favour one side, then the other; go deep, go shallow. I rotate my hips like Elvis. Women are hugely impressed by any guy who doesn't just do that in-out, in-out thing.'
>
> James, 34

Roadtest: 'Jesus! At first I thought, so this is the G-spot, but then I realized it was in a totally different area. It's the only time I've ever come through penetration and is still the only way I can manage it.' *Olivia, 28*

But wait! There's more . . .

The P-spot. It's an area of mucous membrane surrounding the urethral opening and stretching from just below the clitoris to the topof the vaginal opening. Called the 'periurethral glands', researchers think this could be a key area for stimulation during intercourse, perhaps even holding the key to why some women orgasm during penetration alone. Past popular theories say it's because of front wall stimulation, others that these women have bigger than usual clitorises, which are positioned close to the vaginal opening. A study of the P-spot showed that 50 per cent of the area is drawn in and out of the vagina during intercourse on some women, suggesting another possible reason.

Halban's fascia. This is the rather scary name for the space between the bladder and the top wall of the vagina. Packed with collagen and elastin, it not only sounds like a plastic surgery haven, there's also muscle fibre and a rich blood and nerve supply: all ingredients for sensational sexual stimulation.

CAN A WOMAN REALLY EJACULATE LIKE A MAN?

Fifteen years ago, this was a hotly contested topic. Visit your doctor and confess that, 'Umm, sometimes a little bit of liquid comes out when you, umm, you know' and you'll be branded incontinent before you can say, 'Hang on, I really don't think it *is* wee.' These days, most sex researchers assume all women ejaculate, but often in amounts too small to be noticed, even though it's not entirely clear what purpose it serves because the fluid releases too late to act as lubrication.

Ejaculation appears to be linked to the mechanism that closes off the urinary tract during orgasm. If the orgasmic response is super-strong, this closing mechanism can be overcome by the sheer force of orgasmic contractions. This means one or two spurts of urine could be expelled from the bladder quite forcefully, coinciding with orgasmic contractions. However, when analysed, the fluid doesn't have the same make-up as a usual urine sample because it's contaminated by other fluids. Others believe it's not the closing mechanism but periurethral glands surrounding the urethral tube, which are similar to the male prostate. Under extreme stimulation, these glands produce a liquid that's chemically similar to his seminal fluid.

Another popular theory, supported by many of my lesbian friends who claim they and their girlfriends ejaculate on a regular basis, is that ejaculation is linked to the G-spot or a sensitive spot on the front vaginal wall. If the initial theory is true – that it's just a spurt of urine caused

> by a brief relaxation of the bladder muscles after intense
> stimulation and orgasm – this seems about right to me.
> Stimulation of the G-spot initially makes most of us want
> to pee and front wall orgasms are fierce, so it doesn't
> seem too much of a stretch of the imagination to imagine
> the two are linked.

TURN ON TECHNOLOGY:
Sex boosters and erotic elixirs

While there's still no such thing as an aphrodisiac – something which makes anyone turn into an insatiable sexual animal – we're coming pretty close (if you'll excuse the pun). Sex stimulation is a science with researchers inventing all sorts of erotic elixirs, drugs, supplements and devices to help combat most common sexual problems.

Ⓜ FOR HIM

- **Erectile dysfunction drugs:** All three of the main drugs work in the same way: they block an enzyme called PDE5, a chemical which stops erections. There's more PDE5 in the penis than anywhere else in the body and that's why the drugs are so spectacularly successful 'down there'. The biggest misconception about **Viagra** and drugs like it is that they turn *any* man into a walking erection, roaming the streets, mouth frothing, desperate to get a leg-over. Viagra doesn't increase libido at all. If you're not aroused, there's no erection. What they *will* do, is make sure you get a nice, big hard one when there is stimulation, which is, of course, why Viagra is regularly popped for performance enhancement rather than to fix a problem. Bit worried you won't perform for your hot new girlfriend after you've had a few pints? Viagra is a one-night insurance policy that you'll turn on a porn-star performance. Planning on taking a few party drugs but not sure what effect it'll have on later activities? Throwing a little blue pill into the mix seems like a damn good idea, until it lands you in hospital or kills you, that is (cocktail drug combinations are the worst idea you ever had). Again, alarmingly, Viagra has also served to make a frightening number of sexually unsatisfied men visible. The reason sales of Viagra are so unbelievably high, says sex commentator Susie Bright perceptively, is that men see it as a wonder drug which will deliver the sort of sex they think they should have been having all along. 'These are young men (not just older guys looking to recapture their youth) who are finding that sex isn't the mind-blowing, out-of-this-world experience they hoped it would be. And they're humiliated and disappointed that their penises don't always behave themselves so they're turning to Viagra to improve their performance,' Bright says. 'Not only are they disappointed with sex, they also know that if they don't get an erection it won't be pretty – female expectations are pretty high these days.' While it's *not* recommended for anything but the reason it was intended for – erection problems due to blood flow – Viagra has the longest track record for safety and effectiveness. One drawback: food significantly reduces its effectiveness which means that romantic dinner out pre-sex suddenly isn't such a good idea. It's best to wait three hours after a meal before taking a dose and be aware that some men complain of headaches and others of a bluish tint to their vision. **Cialis**, an alternative, can last up to forty-eight hours, which offers the gift of spontaneity. It takes about an hour before you'll get an erection and some suffer a general achy feeling around the back. **Levitra** produces quick erections – within thirty minutes – but again can cause vision problems.

Pre-Viagra, men with erection problems used **vacuum therapy** and it's still a good non-drug, no-side-effect alternative, except that you'd want to be in a long-term relationship or not be easily embarrassed. Vacuum therapy involves using a device that creates a vacuum around the penis, producing an erection by drawing blood into it. The pump is removed, leaving the ring at the base of the penis, which holds the blood in to maintain a firm erection for up to thirty minutes at a time. It takes mere minutes to work, even if you do feel a bit like you're pumping up a spare tyre for your bike rather then getting ready to throw your partner around the bedroom.

> *Nearly half of all UK women have a lower sex drive than they'd like, and almost two thirds would take something like Viagra if it was readily available. The reason for their low libido? Exhaustion.*

- **Delay creams:** Creams or ointments that contain a numbing ingredient can be bought on the internet or in any sex shop. The idea is that if you can't feel as much, you'll be less likely to climax. It's a good concept, but most people don't notice much difference. Not only that, the cream tends to rub off on her as well, which isn't fab when most women have trouble reaching orgasm rather than avoiding it.
- **Testosterone boosters:** A man's testosterone levels drop around the age of forty, and continue to drop by roughly 15 per cent each decade. Since it's the hormone

responsible for maintaining a healthy sex drive in both men and women, this isn't great news. On the other hand, if you're a competitive, aggressive little bugger, you'll become less so when your levels drop. If you're worried, visit your doctor and get your levels checked, then choose from a pill, a patch or a shot. There are side-effects, especially to do with your prostate, which will need to be checked first, and by supplying testosterone it's thought your body will be even less inspired to produce its own.

F FOR HER

- **Viagra** works in a similar fashion for women as it does men: the drug increases blood flow to the clitoris, vaginal lips and vaginal walls. Again, it's not a libido enhancer, so while the flesh may be willing, the mind might not. One study by the US Berman twins, one a psychologist, the other a urologist, found that 67 per cent of women said their ability to have an orgasm increased after taking Viagra and more than 70 per cent said they felt more sensation in the genital area generally.

- **Testosterone boosters:** Slap on a testosterone patch or rub some cream into your forearm and you could notice significant improvements in your sex drive and enjoyment of sex generally. I know several women over fifty who use it and rate it highly. There are side-effects, like increased hair growth, which isn't ideal, but given the choice between waxing or plucking *more* often or having sex *less* often, I know what I'd choose.

- **Hormone replacement therapy (HRT)** is another option. Hormone levels of oestrogen, testosterone and others are measured and balanced. It's a controversial treatment and some say the side-effects are risky, but again it has lots of support and fans.

- **Eros therapy:** This is a small, handheld, battery-operated appliance. It's designed to enhance sexual satisfaction by increasing sensitivity and so improving lubrication to generally up your chances of orgasm. You place a soft cup over the clitoris and turn the device on, creating a gentle vacuum (much like his vacuum therapy). This increases the blood flow to the clitoris and genitals and conditions sensitive tissues leading to genital engorgement. In a Boston study, manufacturers claim 33 per cent of women with normal sexual functioning noticed extra lubrication, 58 per cent increased clitoral sensations, 33 per cent found it easier to orgasm and 25 per cent enjoyed greater sexual satisfaction. I've found response to it divided: some women think it's fabulous, but a few sex therapists I know don't rate it at all.

As more women become financially independent, they're less interested in how much a man earns and more interested in what he looks like. Sound familiar? That's right, it's exactly how wealthy men tend to pick women.

- **Pelvic toners:** These are devices designed to help you exercise the muscles that support the pelvic floor and are crucial for good sex. These range from hard plastic dildos you insert and squeeze your muscles around to something that looks like a spaghetti server with springs, which you squeeze shut and push open again.

Age, childbirth, not having sex often enough and declining oestrogen all have an effect on vaginal muscle tone and continence. I know I'm always raving on about them but doing daily pelvic floor exercises is the single most important thing you can do to ensure a good sex life.

- **Vaginal dilators** are a good self treatment if intercourse is painful because of vaginismus, when your vaginal muscles spasm and close, stopping you from having it. You start with the smallest dilator and work up to penis size, inserting it and consciously squeezing and relaxing your PC muscle at the same time. It works well to overcome the PC spasm reflex.
- **Triphasic birth control pills** have been found to boost sexual interest in women. These pills differ from the standard pill because they have varied progestin levels. The result: women report more sexual interest, fantasies, arousal during sex and sexual satisfaction.
- **Androgen supplements:** If levels of androgen run low, desire drops. Supplements are available and help with both arousal and lubrication.
- **ArginMax:** This is a nutritional supplement – one formula for men and one for women – which you take for several weeks to boost your naturally produced 'sex' hormones. Some notice a marked difference, but not everyone does. Buy it at good health food shops.
- **Scent therapy:** Scentuelle is a patch impregnated with aromas known to have an effect on libido. You slap it on your wrist and smell it frequently during the day to trigger sexual feelings. It's an olfactory approach to female hypoactive sexual desire disorder with 50 per cent of women in the first trial finding it increased their sex drive.

THE G-SHOT: CAN YOU INJECT SUPER SEX?

Fancy bigger, better, more intense orgasms and have half an hour to spare? If you live in LA (where else?) the

solution could simply be to pop along to your local G-shot clinic, dutifully open your legs and your wallet, and let a nice man in a white coat fiddle about a bit, then inject you deep inside your vagina. Yes really. The latest fad, G-spot enhancement, is supposed to increase the sensitivity of your G-spot by plumping it up with collagen, also making it bigger and easier to find. Given that a) not everyone's convinced the G-spot even exists and b) if it does exist, it's only apparent when women are highly aroused, it's going to take a leap of faith and a damn sexy doctor for this to work. But according to the inventor, Dr David Matlock, it's not quite as daft as it sounds. Doctors have used injections of collagen to assist bladder control since the 1940s because it strengthens the area injected.

Patients are left alone to find their own G-spots before a nurse confirms the location, then in strides Dr Matlock, needle in hand. The injection itself takes eight seconds and the effect lasts up to four months. Dr Matlock claims he's had 'ferociously positive' feedback and that the process is virtually risk-free. Well, that's his story anyway.

Listen, I'm not adverse to giving Mother Nature a helping hand and I'm obviously all for more intense orgasms, I just don't think a bit of collagen's going to do it somehow.

5 Sorting Sex Dilemmas

Solutions for when your heart and other parts can't agree

• •

Alas, love does not guarantee great sex, which is why this chapter is devoted to exploring those irritating moral dilemmas like 'Does sex in another country count?' (yes), 'Should I leave if the sex is no good?' (maybe) and 'I some- times fantasize that the fish in my aquarium are sexy mermaids. Should I confess to my partner?' (definitely not because she, like me, will think you're a total loony). While I can't make decisions for you – only *you* know all the individual quirks that make your relationship unique – I can promise to give you lots to think about. And think you must.

The first step to handling moral dilemmas in an adult fashion is to make well thought through decisions rather than hasty, spur-of-the-moment (drunken) ones. This means not putting yourself in a situation where you're horizontal, your pants are around your ankles, brain is floating in a vat of G&T and Mr or Ms Deliciously Tempting (several of them, in fact) are moving in for the kill. Call me sceptical, but I don't believe it's possible to think logically when this is happening. If you really want to do the right thing by your partner – and most

CAN YOU HAVE TOO MUCH SEX?

While most of us shudder at the thought of being addicted to something like heroin, the thought of being addicted to sex is downright appealing. If the government supplies methadone to help heroin addicts kick the habit, surely they'd throw some shiny new sex toys our way or grant 'sex days' instead of 'sick days'? Sigh. But how much is too much and how would we qualify? I counselled a couple on the programme *Hotter Sex*, who claimed they had intercourse around seven times a day, every day. He was home on disability leave: a back problem which strangely prevented him from working in an office but didn't seem to bother him while performing position no. 358 from the *Kama Sutra*. She was a stay-at-home mum who quickly assured me all the activity happened while the kids were at school. Lots of couples diddle the figures when asked how often they have sex, but I believed this pair. They were so damn happy it had to be true. But would I consider them addicted to sex? No. It was enhancing, rather than interfering with their lives and causing no-one any problems (except a spot of jealousy from me and the envious crew).

Sex addiction, like all addictions, puts a destructive twist on an everyday, normal enjoyable activity. Addicts lack the ability to control or postpone sexual feelings and actions. Spending an entire meeting dreaming of getting fellatio from the pretty colleague sitting next to you is not sex addiction. Popping out to make a quick call to a sex worker and arranging for them to service you in the toilets during 'coffee break' is. Sex addicts get to the point where they're willing to risk their relationships, career, even personal health and safety in order to satisfy an insatiable urge. ➤

How do people become sex addicts? Many report abuse or neglect as children or have parents who were also sex addicts. Treatment often includes following a simple change model like the one adopted by Alcoholics Anonymous.

of us do – make a pact not to deliberately put yourself in the path of temptation by going drinking with someone you desperately, desperately lust after. That's just asking for it.

Infidelity aside, there are still other complicated quandaries awaiting the most innocent of couples. Hopefully this will help you tiptoe through the landmines and make it to the other side.

SHOULD YOU STAY IF THE SEX IS NO GOOD?

Some scenarios are fixable. Technique can be taught if you're willing to school a new lover in what you like, where and when. Ignorance about sex in general and a lack of understanding of how your sexual systems work is solved by buying them some good sex books as a present. Harder, but also changeable, are things like reshaping someone's attitude to sex. If they've been brought up to believe sex is bad or dirty, they may need counselling to reshape their deeply ingrained beliefs, but it can still be done. Even dramatically different sex drives can be balanced if you're willing to compromise. It's not such good news if you don't think your partner's a good lover because there's no spark or fireworks – if it's not there in the

37 per cent of UK men agree sex can't be satisfying for women without orgasm. 28 per cent of women agree that sex without orgasm isn't really satisfying for them.

beginning, it's unusual for chemistry to kick in later on. But the only thing which is truly impossible is transforming a selfish, brutish lover into a good or even acceptable one. These people will fight you, kicking and screaming every step of the way. So if you – poor you! – end up with someone like this, I strongly suggest you extradite yourself from the situation ASAP. If your partner is well intentioned, just not terribly good at sex, stay.

DO THOSE DODGY SEX DREAMS MEAN ANYTHING?

Experts tend to divide sharply on the topic of dream analysis. Some claim dreams are simply our sub-conscious trying to make sense of the day, others say they're our way of expressing stifled emotions. Dream interpreters do agree on one thing though: it's often your reaction to what's happening that's most important. If you dream of having sex in public and are lapping up the attention with Mariah Carey-like fervour rather than whimpering with embarrassment, it's likely you're craving attention in real life. No-one truly knows whether dream analysis is a load of old bollocks or a window into our subconscious, but do we really care when it's such good fun analysing the sordid little suckers? These are the most likely interpretations for the most common sex dream scenarios.

Sex with a celebrity: You might present yourself as an innocent, unassuming little thing, but secretly you're an exhibitionist. Dreaming of sex with a celebrity usually means you want to be noticed and crave more glamour.

Dreaming of having a penis (when you don't have one in real life): Constantly having to prove yourself in a male world? It's more likely to be this than good old-fashioned penis envy.

Sex with someone who repulses you in real life: This ➤

---

is often a sign you're still searching for your ideal lover. In our dreams, we're not bound by whether someone's our 'type', so we're freer to explore all the options.

Sex with a stranger: Pay attention to this one. It can mean you're not getting your innermost needs met and are searching for guidance and direction.

Seducing your boss or someone in authority: Authority figures represent control and power and this often means you'd like to take charge in bed. (And the reason you aren't is . . .?) It could also mean you want more power in real life and/or your sex life.

Super-kinky sex with your partner: This one's quite literal – you're keen to try new, adventurous sex but not yet at the point where you're ready to ask for it.

You and your best friend are having sex: It doesn't mean you're secretly lusting after them, but it could mean you're looking for love, approval or understanding from an old friend.

Lusty dreams about your ex: Think about how your ex made you feel. Chances are *that's* what you're missing, rather than him or her.

❶ *Bet you didn't know . . . Sex figures in only about 5 per cent of women's dreams, but when it does, it tends to be shocking and explicit.*

THE SEXLESS MARRIAGE: SHOULD YOU LEAVE IF YOU AREN'T GETTING ANY?

It depends on what else is happening in the relationship, how important sex is to you and whether your partner intends doing something about it. It also depends on how long you've gone without regular sex and if there's a good reason why. If you're both young and healthy but you've spent four of your five years of marriage locked in a bathroom clutching a ratty erotic magazine and having to DIY, you're more than justified in feeling peeved. If your wife has just had a child and you haven't had sex for two months, you're panicking unnecessarily – it's on hold, not gone for ever, promise!

> 'My partner asked me what I was dreaming about because I'd been moaning in my sleep. I was too embarrassed to tell him I'd actually had a nocturnal orgasm while dreaming about having sex with a girl I used to share a flat with.'
>
> Lisa, 38

Sadly, marriage itself is sometimes to blame for a sorry sex life because we often don't marry the people we click with sexually. We'll happily attach our lips and hips to that the pretty-but-dumb person for a five-week fling, but we choose long-term lovers for different reasons. Factors like kindness, stability, intelligence and emotional intelligence take precedence. Which is all terribly sensible but sexual attraction is fundamental: if it's not there, it's not there. The best you can do in that situation is acknowledge that and decide whether you can live with it. If your partner is a good friend and/or brilliant mother or father, you might consider having little or no sex a fair trade. A rich fantasy life and lots of masturbatory sessions might be enough for you. Or you might decide to take a lover, as they do in some European countries, and have your sexual needs satisfied outside the marriage. Or you might decide it's more honest to leave and find someone who does it both ends: for your heart and groin.

You had great sex in the beginning but now it's all disappeared? The first thing to examine before packing your bags is your relationship outside the bedroom. Sex is often used as a bargaining tool, and it could be you're being denied it because your partner is angry with you. Women, especially, are much more likely to lose interest in sex if they're annoyed with their partner. Your relationship's just fine? My next question is this: have you talked about it and admitted it's a problem? There are lots of reasons why you may not have. Saying it out loud – 'Honey, I'm concerned because we haven't had sex for eighteen months' – makes the problem real. You're both then forced to face up to it and (shock horror) *do* something about it, maybe even get (ohmigod, surely not) *help*! Taking yourselves off to see a sex therapist or counsellor is not a sign that your marriage is failing, by the way, it's a sign that you love each other and want your relationship to be as good as it can possibly be. If there's no swinging from chandeliers because *he* doesn't want sex, it's even more unlikely that you've brought it out into the open. All men are sex fiends, after all – well, at least according to urban myth.

Love snuggling up and watching telly in bed? It might be at the expense of your sex life. Italian scientists found that couples who have a TV in their bedroom have sex half as often as those who don't. This is especially true for couples over fifty.

The truth is, there are as many women staring solemnly at the ceiling as their partner turns to face the wall. Lots of sex experts believe low sexual desire in men is America's best-kept secret and the situation in Britain is likely to be the same.

Once you start talking it will become, often painfully, obvious what your future holds. This is the bit when you find out if your partner is willing to work with you to build a satisfying sex life or has no interest in trying to solve the situation. If it's the former, it's great news. You've taken the first, huge step to solving the problem, and in chapter six you'll find all the practical advice you need to take it further. If it's the latter, even the most faithful, supportive partner is forgiven for thinking about leaving – or having a bit on the side. As one therapist puts it: there's something very wrong with the picture if your partner says, 'I know you're desperately unhappy but I don't plan on doing anything about it and I still expect you to be faithful.'

If you've ever wondered, *How come that couple are breaking up, they were perfect together.* Lack of sex is often to blame. It's what you don't see – a marital bed which has become a private hell of avoidance or rejection – that's their undoing. A relationship stripped of the intimacy and physical closeness sex provides feels hollow because the person who's supposed to find you attractive, sexy and desirable doesn't. Who wants to live with that? It's rare for lustless lovers to live happily ever after in platonic bliss. Invariably, one person *isn't* happy in a sexless marriage and ends up either leaving or having an affair.

> 'I counted up the number of times my wife had given me oral sex since we got married seven years ago. Five. We have intercourse about once a month but she makes it very clear it's a chore. I don't know why I stay.'
>
> Alan, 34

DOES SEX WITH AN EX COUNT AS CHEATING IF YOU'VE ALREADY DONE IT BEFORE?

Of course it bloody does, and it can have disastrous consequences for all involved. *You* might be having sex simply because you fancy a bit, and it doesn't feel like you're being unfaithful because it's not someone new, but *they're* often having sex with you in a desperate bid to rekindle the relationship. That means you have to break it off (again) and explain to your current partner why you're suddenly getting plaintive text messages from Deborah/ David after all this time. If you get found out – and the chances of this are higher than if you'd had sex with a ➤

'The only way I can have an orgasm with my boyfriend is to fantasize that he's my ex. It's weird because I don't even like my ex and I love my boyfriend, but I definitely had better sex with him.'

Jenny, 26

IS MONOGAMY TOO MUCH TO EXPECT THESE DAYS?

Not so long ago, Will Smith reputedly told an interviewer if he really fancied someone, he'd say to his wife Jada, 'Look, I need to have sex with somebody. I'm not going to do it if you don't approve of it, but please approve.' Despite this being rather hastily and vehemently denied at a later date, the world seized on the comment as an excuse to air the old 'open marriage vs monogamy' debate and I was asked to comment. Being the jealous type and a tad idealistic I tend to err on the side of monogamy, even though it's clearly an imperfect model for marriage and/or relationships. There's a pathetically hopeful side of me that clings to the concept that we really can only want to have sex with one person. And if that's not true, at least let's pretend guys! Some people do manage it and statistics prove we're faithful more than we're unfaithful. 'So you're against open marriage but you can see monogamy isn't working,' said one journalist. 'What's the solution?' Hmmm. Can I come up with a strategy for world peace instead?

Here's the thing: there's never going to be a perfect solution, because there's no such thing as a perfect one-size-fits-all model for a relationship. Each couple has to come up with a version that suits them. We all have different tastes in clothes, food, cars, houses, travel destinations. We accept that lying on a deserted island is one person's idea of heaven and another's idea of hell. Why can't we accept that while one person will remain happily faithful for forty years, others find it impossible to curb their appetite for the new and exciting? Just as one person climbs into the warm, secure lap of marriage, snuggling and snuffling with contentment, another person frantically clambers out of it, suffocating and gasping for air.

❶ *Couples married for more than thirty years are now twice as likely to divorce as they were ten years ago. Analysts believe this is because women now feel more financially independent.*

At this point, I'd dearly love to sit you both down, tell you to sharpen your pencils and fill in a questionnaire I prepared earlier. You'd then simply tick the boxes, add up your scores and *presto!* your very own model for fidelity. Unfortunately, this is one of those easier-said-than-done exercises. It takes supreme guts or tremendous stupidity to admit you'd like an open relationship without knowing what your partner wants. Admitting you'd prefer monogamy is less traumatic since it's the norm, but sometimes

'I've never been monogamous, promised monogamy or expected it of my partner. I suppose I'm only young, but I just don't see really how it can benefit either of you.'

Carl, 24

you're still not sure if they've got their fingers crossed, desperately hoping you'll opt for regular orgies with anyone who'll say yes. But if you've been going out for a while and it looks like you'll continue to, it could be time for that little chat.

If you're a fan of open relationships, be aware that plenty of people assume you'll be monogamous if nothing is said to the contrary. Then again there are people who'll feign innocence if caught cheating, saying you hadn't actually agreed to forsake all others. Cover all bases by clearly, firmly and specifically spelling out what it is you expect from your partner. Remember, there aren't just two options, some of the alternatives are listed below. Think outside the box and, of course, practice safe sex if you do opt to be with other people.

Looking for a partner who's guaranteed not to cheat? According to a world expert, they should be religious, have friends who support monogamy, live in a small community, have parents and grandparents who haven't even dreamed of being unfaithful, work alone, close to home and never travel for business. Suddenly prepared to take a bit of a risk? I'm with you!

Monogamy

You only have sex and/or intimate contact with your partner.

Points to negotiate: What does 'intimate' contact involve? Flirting, kissing, heavy petting, oral sex, intercourse? Where is the line drawn? (See 'Are You an Emotional Cheat?', pages 168–171)

What's great about it: You both feel special, knowing you're committed to an intimate, exclusive relationship. This model is the norm, so it feels comfortable for most people, offering stability and security.

What's not so great: It's not nicknamed 'monotomy' for nothing. Lots of couples get bored having the same sexual partner for life. It is possible to have great long-term sex, but you do need to work at it.

Attempted monogamy

You both try your best to be monogamous but agree to turn a blind eye to one-night stands or slip-ups that aren't pre-meditated. Nothing is done that will embarrass each other, i.e. no sex with mutual friends or acquaintances or confessing to other people.

Points to negotiate: Do you want to know about these slip-ups? Is there a limit to how many per year/five years/ten years?

What's great about it: This is an increasingly common solution to balancing the pros and cons of monogamy. It shows a strong desire to do the right thing but also allows for human error. It's realistic but not completely unromantic.

What's not so great: You need to be mature and secure to get your head around this. If you're the jealous type, you won't be able to resist constantly checking to see if anything has happened. It also requires a high level of trust to accept your that partner really will only use the escape clause as a last resort.

An open relationship with limits

You both agree you'll have sex with other people but there are rules.

Points to negotiate: Who's allowed, who's not? Are you allowed to sleep with a person more than once? Do you want to be told?

What's great about it: You get the security of having a long-term partner but the freedom to enjoy the thrill of new partners. Couples who don't believe in 'owning' each other tend to opt for this one and it works well for gay men.

What's not so great: Most people are black and white about open relationships and feel strongly one way or another. The majority don't believe they work and will be offended if you even suggest it. Quite often, one partner wants this type of relationship while the other wants monogamy, but agrees to it simply because they know their partner will leave if they don't. If you're jealous or traditional in your views, it's definitely not for you.

'Open' or 'closed' swinging

You both have sex with other people, either in front of each other (open) or privately (closed).

Points to negotiate: How far do you want to take it? Kissing, touching, oral, intercourse? Which activities are allowed, which aren't?

What's great about it: It's a good solution for couples who can't cope with an open relationship but feel suffocated and unfulfilled just sleeping with one person. Swinging tends to be controlled, in that you usually do it together. Some people see it as an honest way to sleep around and it's becoming more popular.

What's not so great: If you're in love, most people can't cope with the thought of their partner having sex with someone else, let alone actually watching it happen.

An open relationship

You are both free to sleep with whoever you want, whenever you want.

Points to negotiate: In a true open relationship anything goes, but most couples set a few ground rules specific to their situation.

> **50 per cent of over forty-fives who participated in Durex's 2006 Global Sex Survey admitted to having had an affair.**

What's great about it: If you're highly sexed, not in the slightest bit possessive and enjoy multiple partners, this is probably your idea of sexual nirvana. It's usually chosen by couples with high libidos and open minds and is worth giving a try if it truly is what you both want.

What's not so great: I've only met two long-term couples in the whole time I've been writing and researching sex who are genuinely happy with this arrangement. It works if you're young and not ready to settle down or not particularly attached to your partner, but is fraught with all sorts of obvious problems for everyone else.

I HAD AN AFFAIR BUT NOW IT'S OVER. MUST I COME CLEAN TO SAVE THE RELATIONSHIP?

It depends very much on the circumstances. If the affair is known or strongly suspected, you're usually better off telling. You won't gain by denying it because you'll probably get found out anyway and you might save the relationship by confessing. As the late US psychologist Shirley Glass, generally recognized as the world expert on infidelity, said, 'Marriages fare better after a voluntary confession than after an unwanted discovery'. Another time to tell is if you're in therapy because your relationship is in trouble. There's virtually no point in going if you're not going to confess to an affair. The whole point of therapy is to provide a nice, safe environment (free of rolling pins and heavy objects) where you can both tell the truth and sort out issues once and for all. If you've agreed to therapy because you're planning on leaving but feel obliged to trot along before doing so, call the therapist and explain the situation privately.

But there are also valid reasons for keeping your mouth shut. If your partner's bullying you into a confession with one hand poised to pull the pin on a hand grenade, lie your ass off. Confession also means you'll be living with someone who sees you as less than perfect, and many ➢

people can't cope with that. The *New Yorker* ran a fabulous cartoon featuring a sad-looking man drowning his sorrows at a bar, with the caption, 'My wife understands me.' Our looking-glass selves – other people's opinions of us reflected back – influence our self-perception. If you don't like the person you see in their eyes, you won't like yourself much either. Some experts will also advise you not to tell if your partner's not the strongest person emotionally because news of an affair isn't exactly going to give them a leg up on that steep, bumpy road to high self-esteem. Telling is going to wipe out any trust they *had* managed to muster, and it could take years to rebuild (if, indeed, that's possible at all). Whether you decide to kiss and tell or not, the most important thing is to establish is why you had the affair in the first place. What were you getting from it that you aren't getting from the relationship you're in, and is it possible to create that with the person you're already with?

F FOR HER

SEVEN REASONS WHY YOU'RE TEMPTED TO CHEAT ON YOUR BOYFRIEND (AND WHY NOT ONE OF THEM IS WORTH IT)

The bleak truth is that even the purest of us are tempted by certain situations or people and almost everyone is susceptible to the grass-is-greener syndrome. Even if you've got no intention of actually being unfaithful, you might still find yourself wistfully pulling on your stockings instead of pop socks for that 'innocent' drink. You have no intention of him ever seeing them – God forbid, your guilty self assures you – but there's nothing wrong with a healthy fantasy life, eh? Indeed. But just in case you are tempted to move the play from your head to your bed, be warned: in most classic temptation situations, you might find you're not missing out on a thing . . .

1. I can tell him things I can't tell my boyfriend

Why you might be tempted: He's the guy at work/the gym who you're just starting to get to know. At first it's just chit-chat, but one day you reveal something quite personal and he's so understanding and supportive you're amazed. Much more understanding, you think grumpily, than my boyfriend, and he's *supposed* to care. So the chats become more personal and more frequent and before long you're thinking, 'maybe this person understands me more, he feels like my soulmate'. Seduced by the wondrous feeling of being able to bare your soul without fear of judgement, you forget the reason why you can be so open: if you don't meet with this man's approval, so what? You've got little invested in the relationship and therefore little to lose.

Why it wouldn't be worth it: Many people find it easier to bare their soul to a stranger than the partner they've known for more than a decade. Why? Our partner already has a perception of us and we're aware that confessing certain things may alter that, so we censor our conversations, usually without being aware of it. Talk of sex with anyone else – pre-them or a current wistful daydream – is banned and since most of us have made some sort of future commitment to a partner, so is vocalizing those wacky but oh-so-appealing fantasies of taking a year off and trekking through Cambodia/chucking in your job to go back to uni. The joy of talking openly and honestly with someone who's only known us for a short time can be incredibly intoxicating, but it doesn't mean you should cheat or leave your current boyfriend for them. The minute *he* becomes

> **People who expect their partners to betray them will usually do it themselves first.**

your boyfriend, the same rules will apply. Be careful with this one: we are closest to the people who know the most about us, and those 'innocent' chats can cause major damage long term.

2. He listens, my boyfriend doesn't

Why you might be tempted: If unashamedly baring your soul feels good, imagine someone who listens to you, and I mean *really* listens to you – even when you're talking utter rubbish. When you talk to your boyfriend, his eyes remain fixed on the telly or you can see his fingers itching to turn the page of the paper. When you talk to *this* guy, you get 150 per cent complete, undivided attention. This makes you feel important, heard, understood, attracted . . . and tempted.

> **One study found that men who cheat tend to be sociable and outgoing while women who play away are often needy and withdrawn. This fits with the theory than men are opportunistic and women cheat when they're unhappy.**

Why it wouldn't be worth it: The ability to find stories of how traumatic it was when your goldfish died completely fascinating tends to wear off around the six-month mark. Even then, it's not the story they're listening to; they're watching your face, your hands, your eyes, your expressions (your breasts) lost in the wonderment of *you*. Sadly, the kick-ass love hormones responsible for this highly addictive 'glorifying' eventually drop off and completely dry up after eighteen months. Then suddenly you're not quite so entertaining. 'I didn't feel heard' is the No. 1 reason cited by women filing for divorce, and it's not a pleasant feeling. Happily, though, there's lots you can do to stop being and feeling ignored.

First up, work out what it is you want to say. Men are literal and direct, women tend to plonk a lot of detail and emotion on top which can mean the message gets lost. He may be lazy and not making an effort, or he might have turned off because most of your talking is actually (dare I say) boring. Is what he's ignoring worth listening to? We make more effort to be entertaining with others than we do with our long-term partners. Your new infatuation is nodding and

❶ *If you think your partner is being unfaithful and you're female, you're probably right. One of New York's top private eyes claims women's instincts are usually spot on.*

gazing with rapt attention because you're telling a genuinely funny story. Possibly the same funny story that had your current boyfriend guffawing and slapping his leg with amusement not so long ago.

3. My boyfriend's getting a bit boring in bed. I bet this guy wouldn't be

Why you're tempted: Intellectually we know being in love with someone doesn't mean we stop fancying other people, but there's a tiny, hopeful, ridiculously idealistic part of all of us that secretly believes if we're with the *right* man, this won't happen. So it comes as quite a shock when, usually around two years in, you meet someone who does it for you – again. They start creeping into your thoughts, your fantasies and suddenly they're in your bed as you make love to your boyfriend while guiltily wishing it was him instead. You're a staunch supporter of fidelity and have no real intention of acting on it but . . . everyone else seems to be doing it, so maybe it's not such a big deal any more? Would it really hurt anyone if you just kissed him? Who would know?

Why it wouldn't be worth it: Even if it doesn't lead to anything more (yeah right), you don't give into the irresistible pleasure of telling close friends (ditto), they don't tell others (fact: people tell at least one other person a secret they've promised to keep) and he doesn't end up finding out (easier than you think), the bottom line is *you'd* know you'd done it. You'd lose respect for yourself, him and the relationship because you've broken the trust bond. We all crave the luscious, lusty sex you get at the beginning of a relationship, but it can quickly get lost in daily life. It's hard work keeping sex fresh and exciting when you've decided to make love to just one person for the rest of your life. But it can be done and the payoff is a level of fulfilment light years away from the pleasure of one hot night with a stranger. Of course this man seems much more appealing: he's new, unexplored territory. Swap him for your current boyfriend and you'll be swapping *him* for someone else when the boredom kicks in again. And again. And again.

> ❶ *Women with red hair have more sex, according to a study of hundreds of German women. If your partner decides to dye her hair that colour, watch out: it's likely she's looking for someone better.*

4. I have more fun with him than I do my boyfriend

Why you're tempted: He's a friend of your brother's, a client of the company, the guy in the next flat. You've struck up a friendship and you're thoroughly enjoying it because he's funny. He makes you laugh – and humour is something that's in short supply with your boyfriend these days. All you seem to do with him is talk about mundane things. It's whose turn is it to do the dishes vs someone who makes you feel light-hearted, giggly and carefree. Is it any wonder you're feeling peeved and more than a little curious about what might happen if you took it further.

Why it wouldn't be worth it: The chances of you ending up in exactly the same position a few years in with your new man are even higher than the likelihood of me wandering into the kitchen in the next two minutes to make a cup of coffee. We like to think we're individual, but most couples hit the same set of problems around the same time. A major, common hiccup is that the relationship moves from fun to functional. This starts the second you decide to get serious about each other because you don't just get serious about your feelings, you get serious about life. Those long, boozy Sunday lunches that always ended up with the two of you in bed get replaced by flat-hunting, decorating and working overtime to keep up the mortgage payments. But that flat, no matter how fabulous, isn't what's going to keep you together. It's the weekends away, holidays, nights out together having fun that will guarantee you stay in love.

5. I argue with my boyfriend all the time, but never with him

Why you're tempted: You're starting to feel a bit like Cathy and Heathcliff from *Wuthering Heights* given all the dramatic arguments, slamming doors and stomping about at home. In comparison, being with your friend Mark feels blissfully stress free. With him, you can say/do/wear/watch whatever you want, without fear of offending or being offended. Home feels like a battlefield and time with your best male friend is fast becoming your sanctuary.

Why it wouldn't be worth it: Of course you're not going to argue with a male friend; you've got nothing to argue about. You're (hopefully) not having sex, you're not sharing a house and you're not having to negotiate and juggle the demands of housework, friends and everyday life. We're far more on our best behaviour with our friends than our partners. Besides, arguments are healthy: they show you're secure enough to question each other's beliefs and behaviour. They also show you care what your partner thinks and feel passionate enough about them to want to fight to change their opinions or behaviour. According to relationship guru John Gottman, so long as you're having five good times to every one bad time, your relationship is in a healthy state. It's the couple who *don't* argue who need to worry. There's a fine line between love and hate but topple over into indifference and you're really in trouble. Assuming the arguments with your boyfriend aren't physically or emotionally abusive and you come up with solutions, you could both simply have volatile personalities which secretly thrive on drama.

6. My boyfriend never compliments me, this guy treats me like a princess

Why you're tempted: A final daub of gloss, earrings that cost more than you care to admit, and we won't even talk about the shoes. Studying yourself in the mirror, even you're impressed with the result. You teeter down the stairs to present the ultra-glam you to your partner and he looks up and says . . . absolutely nothing. Terrific. So you flounce out the door to your work do and the guy from the office you mildly flirt with all the time sees you and says, 'Wow!', then he spends the whole night following you around telling you how beautiful and clever you are, and how if *he* was your boyfriend he wouldn't let you out of his sight. We're all a little narcissistic, thriving on the high of being worshipped, so who could blame you for gravitating toward flattery?

Why it wouldn't be worth it: If you're in this situation, it's usually a case of new love versus old: the tried-and-true up against the new and infinitely more exciting. You're confused, and with good reason. Love feels very different at different stages in your relationship. New love is excitement, old love is contentment: the long sigh that escapes when you're snuggled by the fire, watching a DVD while eating fish and chips. Both are equally as appealing, but in wildly different ways. The new person treats you like a princess because he's trying to woo you. He's showering you with compliments and giving you 100 per cent attention because it's early days. It's what your current boyfriend did in the beginning too, remember, and it's what he might do again if you pointed out how much you miss it. Be warned: most relationships seem promising in the first few months, but few make it past that.

SHOULD YOU LEAVE IF HE CAN'T GIVE YOU AN ORGASM?

It's one thing ditching a man who makes absolutely no attempt to find out why you haven't climaxed or tried to rectify the situation, but it's quite another to dump a guy who spends every waking hour desperately devouring sex manuals and has practically dislocated his tongue trying to make it happen. Quite honestly, no man can *give* you an orgasm, you have to take one for yourself. That means learning how to orgasm through using a vibrator or masturbation, then showing him how to do it with his fingers. You then need to direct him how to use his tongue, and explain that you need certain positions – ones that hit the front vaginal wall – or an extra hand, finger or vibrator to help you climax during intercourse. All this puts the responsibility for orgasm back on you. Which is where it should be: it's your body and your orgasm. You have to speak up and communicate what it is you need to tip you over. Sure, there are some men out there who are such experienced lovers they'll magically hit on a technique that does it for you. But being a good lover doesn't mean he'll be a great partner, and leaving a man who can't give you an orgasm because he doesn't have a clue what you need ➢

7. My boyfriend's not going anywhere and this guys a real go-getter.

Why you're tempted: You've just changed jobs and suddenly you're mixing with a completely different type of man than you're used to. Your boyfriend's got a perfectly good job but he's not exactly going to set the world on fire – unlike Jake. He's the head of the new team you're working with and he's put the *Cor!* into corporate. He also pays you lots of attention, hinting at a lifestyle you find intoxicatingly exciting. Life with him would never be dull, you catch yourself thinking.

Why it wouldn't be worth it: You're right, life with this new guy probably wouldn't be dull, but it might be upsetting, unsettling and heartbreaking. The downside of hooking up with a high-achiever is that their job often comes first, second, third and fourth; they work long hours, with little time left for you, and tend to travel a lot with plenty of cash to splash on whoever they'd like to share that posh hotel room with. As their partner, you're required to tag along to all those company dinners (yawn!) and look the part (no more chocolate forever). High-flyers can also be 'sensation seekers', people who need more excitement and novelty than others to experience any sort of 'high'. Scientists have found that low levels of certain brain chemicals, mainly dopamine and serotonin (responsible for feelings of happiness and contentment), mean some people are more likely to cheat because of the enormous rush that lying and having forbidden sex provides. Yes, he's got the glam car and swollen expense account, but at what cost?

HELP, I FANCY MY GYNAECOLOGIST. IS IT A BIT WEIRD FOR ME TO ASK HIM OUT? IS IT EVEN LEGAL?

And here I was thinking it was just me! After confessing to friends, I discovered that fancying the man brandishing that horrid cold, metal thing is incredibly common, if a little surprising given what he does with it and how uncomfortable the whole situation is. That's why it's absolutely imperative you approach this one with a great deal of thought. For starters, is he even single? Surreptitiously pump the staff for personal info – 'I don't know what I'd do without Dr Green. He's absolutely fantastic! Imagine being his wife, how amazing would that be: all your problems solved on the spot,' then hope like hell they volunteer, 'Wife? He doesn't have one'. Once you've established whether he's available, the next step is to take an objective, rather than hopeful, look at your appointments, looking for any signs of interest on his part. Needless to say the usual giveaways that a guy fancies you – him buying you a drink, 'accidentally' touching you, trying to put his tongue down your throat under the guise of a goodbye kiss – aren't applicable here. Instead, look for subtler signs. Does he lean forward when talking to you? Does he appear to spend longer with you than other patients? Does he steer the conversation away from medical matters to personal stuff? Did you get the feeling he looked sort of pleased when you said you were single? If you're as certain as you can be that there's interest on his part, you've then got little choice but to ask him out. He's not allowed to ask you out, remember, so this *has* to come from you. Word it tactfully and it won't be hugely embarrassing – 'Look I know this is a bit weird given that you're my doctor, but I was wondering if you'd like to get together for a drink ➤

sometime? I really enjoy talking with you'. At this point he will probably say, 'I'm afraid I can't do that. It's not acceptable for doctors to date their patients,' or, '*I'd like to*, but it's not acceptable . . .' If he says 'I'd like to', that's your cue to say, 'Well, I'm sure you could refer me on to someone else if that's a problem.' He agrees and *Voila!* you have a date. Sneaky, eh?

THE NEW INFIDELITY: LOOK BUT DON'T TOUCH AFFAIRS

There's always been an unwritten rule that thou shall not play tonsil-tennis with another person, allow them to put their hands or tongues on your parts or insert their bits into yours. The equation is simple: sex = infidelity. But now cheating has taken on a whole new meaning. Psychologists are saying emotional infidelity – deep, passionate connections between people who often aren't even aware they've crossed the line from platonic friendship to romantic love – is the biggest threat marriage has ever faced.

Infidelity expert Shirley Glass first identified it in her book *NOT "Just Friends"*. She said 82 per cent of the unfaithful partners she'd counselled had an affair with someone who'd started out as a friend. Emotional infidelity wasn't part of our grandparents' consciousness because the only member of the opposite sex available to flirt with was either your best friend's husband or your husband's best friend. Neither are great candidates for a quick fling. As if to prove the theory that familiarity breeds lust, infidelity rose sharply the second

> **Only 46 per cent of men think online affairs count as adultery – but they now cause one third of US divorce litigation.**

women swelled the workforce and expanded the choice of men available to have an affair with. One study showed that 50 per cent of unfaithful women and 62 per cent of unfaithful men were involved with someone at work. Women travelling alone with male co-workers, an increasingly permissive society that condones opposite sex friendships, 'harmless', flirty email banter – it's all now seen as totally acceptable. Except, of course, to the jealous partner left behind or struggling to cope with it all (though usually they're loath to question it for fear of looking hopelessly uncool and old-fashioned).

DOES CHEATING EXIST IF THERE'S NO-ONE AROUND TO CATCH YOU?

You told no-one, there's absolutely no chance you'd ever get found out, you will never see them again, you had safe sex and it meant nothing. Does cheating really matter in that case? It depends totally on your personality. If you genuinely see nothing wrong with what you did and your motivation was solely opportunity, how could it possibly harm your relationship? Your partner is none the wiser and your behaviour towards them hasn't altered. There's just one problem with the perfect infidelity crime: very few people truly believe there's nothing wrong with cheating. Even the smoothest, slickest philanderer, fond of boasting of their conquests to equally slimy friends, is aware that they're doing something wrong. And this is where it all unravels. Knowing we've done something which would hurt our partner subtly alters our perception of them. You got away with something, you're one up on them. This makes them appear either naïve and too trusting or vulnerable and hopelessly helpless. Good relationships ➢

Add to this myriad new, deliciously secret ways to contact our new or old 'friends' – text, email, Friends Reunited, chatrooms and websites catering for every possible sexual whim – and it's no wonder the lines of infidelity have blurred.

Intense but invisible, erotic but unconsumed – emotional infidelity is dangerous, addictive and way too easy to get away with. With the boundaries blurring, it's hard to know what's acceptable and what's not. Are you emotionally unfaithful? Is your partner cheating without ever having laid a hand on someone else? See how you and your partner rate by answering the following questions honestly:

Are you an emotional cheat?

❶ *If your mother or father cheated, the chances are you will, too. A study of more than 2,000 women across the US found 13 per cent of women who'd been unfaithful had five or more affairs and had grown up with a parent who had also been unfaithful.*

- **Do you talk negatively about your partner to a special friend?** Bad-mouth your spouse and you're giving this person the green light to woo you. You're effectively saying, 'I could be lured away from this relationship because it's not ideal'.

- **Do you act available?** I had a highly embarrassing situation recently where I'd just waved off my new boyfriend and popped to the shops. Feeling particularly perky and attractive after an afternoon in bed with him, I noticed a man pulling up on a bike to let me cross the road. Adding an exaggerated swing to my hips as I walked, I flirtily glanced over my shoulder, sending him a smouldering look and cheeky little smile. Once I'd crossed the road, I naughtily looked back again, only to see he'd turned the corner and was following me. Swiftly changing from Ms Could-be-available-if-you-play-your-cards-right to stalker-alert behaviour, I was simultaneously relieved and mortified to discover the man behind the bike helmet was . . . my new boyfriend. 'Oh, it's you,' I said, confused and caught out (I didn't realize he owned a motorbike). 'If you didn't know it was me, why were you being all flirty then?' he quite rightly said. The moral of this cautionary tale: if you're happily involved, don't act single and available.

> **According to research by psychologists, most people believe sending emails late at night and revealing personal details of your life are key signs your partner is having a virtual affair.**

- **Do you have one rule for you, one rule for them?** A gloriously attractive cameraman I worked with was consistently chatted up by women and claimed that for every fifty offers, he only said yes to one. His wife, according to him, was never propositioned, which made him more faithful than she was, given that she was never put in the path of temptation. There's a weird sort of logic there but I'm still not buying it. We all want to have our cake and eat it, but we justify it by saying that dangerous flirtation is innocent. We're also very good at deluding ourselves that something's innocent when it's not because it's such bloody good fun flirting with an attractive someone who isn't your partner.
- **Do you regularly indulge in sexual fantasies about someone else?** This is a tough one. I don't actually think

there's anything intrinsically wrong with being unfaithful in your head, but lots of experts disagree with me and say affairs start in the mind. I do concede that fantasy sex can make you want the person even more. The whole point of fantasies, after all, is to conjure up brilliantly perfect sex. While the real-life encounter is likely to be far less exciting, strong images can make you want something even more.

> 'I find it quite alarming that my sex drive puts me into situations where I really don't want to be. Sometimes it feels like it's in charge of my brain rather than the other way around.'
>
> Tom, 25

- **Do you keep secrets?** Do you have secret email accounts, passwords and a lock on your phone? In an open, honest relationship no communication is a secret. Vow that no text or email will contain anything you don't want your partner to read. If you receive something saucy you haven't solicited, mention it or show it to your partner.
- **Do you share intimate details of your life with people you fancy?** It's one thing dissecting and analysing your relationships with same-sex friends or opposite-sex gay friends, but it's quite another discussing deeply personal issues with someone you've got a 'thing' for. Emotional closeness swiftly moves into romantic dependence.
- **Do you step outside the boundaries/rules you've made as a couple?** All couples have mutually agreed rules, spoken or unspoken, and most people know when they've overstepped the line.
- **Do you lie to your partner about seeing other people?** Your partner's feeling a little threatened by the amount of time you're spending with your new best friend, so you've started pretending you're with other people they trust, because you're fed up with having to explain yourself and it's all innocent anyway. Oh yeah? If it's so innocent, why

are you lying? if your partner really has got a problem with jealousy, encourage them to seek counselling. Otherwise, their jealousy is justified: you're giving too much of yourself and your time to someone else.

> *One in twenty-five British men have no idea they aren't the fathers of the children who call them Daddy.*

Good questions to ask yourself to keep you on the straight and narrow are: if your partner saw you right now, would they be upset? Would you be tempted to lie about what you're doing? If yes, stop it. Similarly, don't have regular contact with a person they don't know about. If you tell your partner about a flirtation or friendship, it usually means you're not going to act on it. Having lunch or dinner three times a week with someone and 'forgetting' to tell your partner about it is tantamount to saying, 'I don't want you to know about this person because I'm not sure where it's all going to lead.'

- **Are you female?** It tends to be the woman who pushes the affair from friendship to love, from fantasy to actuality, according to psychologists. Women get more emotionally involved and are keen to test it out and see if it could be better than their current situation. For most men, affairs – both flirtations and those consummated in the flesh – are high opportunity and low involvement. She's seeing him as her soul mate, he's just having fun.

6 Couple's Climax Clinic

Lust for the long haul

•••

When a book called *How to Make Love to the Same Person for the Rest of Your Life – and Still Love It* was published in 1985, every long-term couple I knew bought a copy within a week. As far as book titles go, this takes some beating. It's compelling, seductive and packed with the promise of what most couples were starting to think didn't exist: long-term sexual happiness. The author, Dagmar O'Connor, wasn't the first to address the problem of the monotony of monogamy, but that title sure as hell got it talked about. Instead of being every couple's guilty little secret, dreary long-term sex became the new dinner party debate.

Years later, we're still talking about it. Partly because it beats having constant conversations about work, kids and sport, but mostly because, for some, 'hot monogamy' is still as elusive as a wet bar of soap in a shower. I'd say most couples hover halfway between bedroom boredom and bliss, but a few smug bastards really have cracked it. Despite the dour picture drawn by the media, long-term doesn't always equate to short on sex.

Headlines like 'The Sexless Marriage' and 'The Sex-Starved Marriage' lead you to believe that sex is happening everywhere except in the marital bed, but most research says – and always has said, by the way – that married couples have more sex, more varied sex and, incidentally, more oral sex than singles. On the other hand, the number of young couples who either don't have sex at all or have it less often than their parents is growing. Brought up to believe they're missing their sexual prime if they're not at it like rabbits in their twenties, these couples are silent sufferers, secretly thinking they must be doomed.

One thing that hasn't changed is this: there are still a lot of myths out there. Like the one that says the best sex we have is when we're young (our genitals may be in peak condition but it takes more than working parts to have great sex) the one that says it's always the woman who doesn't feel like sex (not true, it's about 50/50 – women are just more comfortable with admitting it) and the one that says if you're having sex problems you're on a slippery slope to the end of your relationship. According to top sex therapists, one of the most widespread and destructive myths is that happy couples have a consistent sex life. Almost every couple goes through dry spells; it's the way you react to them which is more telling.

True sexual compatibility is about being able to adapt to each other's sexual preferences – and that's what this chapter is all about. Creating long-term sexual happiness by being flexible, open to change and trying new things. Here you'll find what I think are the most important new theories on long-term lust, some practical solutions to common couple problems, some DIY sex therapy and a lot, lot more.

MAKEOVER YOUR RELATIONSHIP IN ONE WEEKEND

Got no firm plans this weekend? Skip the DVD and takeaway

and instead give your love life a makeover – it might just guarantee you really *do* live happily ever after.

Saturday: your relationship
Find out who you're in love with

Lots of couples talk to each other but few listen properly or without judgement. This exercise teaches you how to do both and is also designed so you can get to know your partner as they are now as opposed to how they were when you first met – because that was probably the last time you allowed each other to talk uninterrupted, without making a comment or silent judgement.

> **Women over forty claim they're having the best sex of their lives and feel more adventurous in bed than they did in their twenties. And it's married women who are having the most fun.**

I've written the instructions from the perspective of the person doing the listening. And yes, this will have to be you at some point, so grit your teeth and volunteer to go first. Also I'm going to be Ms Bossy Boots for this one and insist you follow some rules or it won't work. OK here goes . . .

- **You each get a turn to talk** to the other for half an hour – if this seems too much for either of you, make it fifteen minutes.
- **The person talking can only talk about themselves**, not about you or the relationship. Instead, they should focus generally on their emotions, their needs, what they've learned from books or films they've watched, what they think about their friends, their family, job, what they like about themselves, what they don't, how they're enjoying life and how they're coping.
- **You're not allowed to interrupt** or even comment on

what's been said. Your job is simply to listen and try to understand the person talking.

- **Watch your facial expressions and body language.** Nod supportively, say, 'Uh-huh' and smile encouragingly. Sitting there sulking over something they've said or with a thunderous expression is going to thwart the whole exercise.
- **If you really, really, *really* must comment** on something your partner's said, **wait twenty-four hours**. Then, if you still can't help yourself, you're allowed ten minutes maximum. One other catch: the comments can only be positive. If you think there's a problem, outline it quickly, then spend the rest of the time talking about possible solutions. 'What you said about wanting to spend more time with your friends has made me realize we need to make the most of the time we do spend together,' rather than, 'I can't believe you want to spend more time down the pub with those useless friends of yours, you selfish sod'.
- After doing this exercise **don't be surprised if you both feel a little unnerved**. You've probably just discovered things about your partner you didn't know, and that's why you feel slightly uncomfortable. Who is this person? You thought you knew them inside out – what a shock, eh? You don't own each other and can't control how you both feel, so relax and go with the uncertainty. Taking your partner completely for granted is what kills most relationships. It does both of you good not to feel 100 per cent sure of each other.
- **Repeat this session once a week for a month** and you'll find you start to listen properly without it having to be a structured exercise.

Get exactly what you want

Another classic relationship mistake is assuming that because your partner loves you, they know what you need to make you happy. Sadly, love doesn't magically transform us into mind-readers, so we rely on the next best thing: we assume what makes *us* happy will make *them* happy which, as you can imagine, leads to unmitigated disasters. You get tickets to the cup final for your birthday along with the latest Nintendo game. He gets an inspirational self-help book and dinner in a romantic (i.e. stuffy) restaurant. To completely guarantee a life of misery, we take this warped thinking even further. We assume if our partner doesn't behave the way *we* would in a particular situation, they don't care about us. Cue typical couple arguments about things like anniversaries (some people place importance on them, others don't) chatting up your best friend (seen as charming her by one, flirting by another). Happily, there is a way to fix this sorry situation. It's called being clear about what you both want.

- **For the next month, each of you gets a 'me' day**, taking it in turns until the month is up.
- **On your 'me' day, you get to ask** your partner **for something you'd like** that makes you happy. It might be something as simple as ensuring they turn up on time to pick you up; massaging your shoulders while you're watching telly or holding your hand while walking along.
- **State *clearly* what you'd like your partner to do**, giving as much detail as possible. The idea is to get into the habit of asking for what you need and want to make you happy rather than expecting your partner to second guess.
- **Pay attention to what your partner asks for.** Write down what they requested and you'll have a list of your partner's real needs and wants rather than what you *think* they want or don't want.

Sunday: your sex life
Don't just maintain, nurture
When you start a new relationship, your focus is on your sex life. You're learning about your partner's body with

beginner's lust fuelling your curiosity. When you think you've got each other figured out, most couples move from nurturing their sex life into maintaining it. Six weeks into your relationship, the proportion is around 80 per cent (nurturing) to 20 per cent (maintenance). Six years on it's more like 0 to 100. To keep sex good long term, you have to continue to nurture. This means putting thought and energy into sex, just like you did in the beginning.

- **Take turns with sex-spoil sessions.** Every fifth time you have sex, one of you spoils the other with things you know they enjoy – note the emphasis on what *they* enjoy, not what *you* enjoy! This might be as simple as giving them a gloriously thorough working over with your tongue or involve you packing a picnic to head off for sex alfresco.

- **Take a sexual inventory.** Write suggestions for some new sexual activities on two sheets of paper and take turns rating them from hot (would love to try) to warm, luke-warm and cold (would rather cut off all your fingers and toes). They might include spanking, role play, semi-public sex, tie-up games, blindfolding, talking dirty, anal sex, watching or making erotic films. When you're done, action the activities which scored high for both of you and try one every two weeks or once a month.

Turn your bedroom into a sex den

Sex in a bog-standard bedroom is a yawn. Sex in an erotic, exotic playroom is sexier than that recurring fantasy of your favourite celebrity walking into your bedroom just as you're reaching into the bedside drawer. Some essentials are:

- **Soundproof it** for kids/flatmates/your mother when she comes to stay: Heavy curtains and carpets soak up sound, and if you're deadly serious, install sound-insulating board on any adjoining walls. A lazy but effective option is to put in a sound system or radio. Music masks all sorts.

- **Get the lighting right.** For the most flattering lighting, light from below or at eye level. Dimmers are the next best thing and can match whatever mood you're in. A simple, quick fix in the meantime is to put tea-lights on saucers on the floor, though best to keep them a safe distance from bedcovers or enthusiastically thrown bras, knickers or boxers.
- **Add a mirror.** Mirror wardrobe doors can be angled to provide a good view of the bed or use a full-length portable mirror which you can move into whatever position takes your fancy.

> **It's not who you know, it's who you marry.** New research shows your position in society, measured by income and status, depends mainly on who you marry. Social mobility – whether people remain in the same class and income bracket to which they were born – is mainly explained by marriage.

- **Add toys and essentials.** Massage oil, stockings and scarves for tie-up, sleep masks from your last plane flight to act as a blindfold, lubricant, condoms, erotic books or movies, sexy clothes, vibrators and other sex toys.
- **Check your bed.** A firm bed makes for better sex and clean, fresh, good-quality sheets lure you to lie naked on them. Cushions are a must for putting under hips, supporting limbs or making other places around the house sex-friendly.
- **Install a bidet.** They might look old-fashioned and out of date, but they're perfect for freshening up before, during or after sex.

ARE YOU TOO CLOSE FOR GREAT SEX?

It's ironic that the couples who have the closest, soul-mate connection and the best relationships often have the worst sex lives. Why? Because the same achingly wonderful intimacy that makes us yearn to merge as one obliterates desire by completely neutralizing sexual chemistry. Almost anyone who's ever been in love subliminally senses the point when the relationship subtly but significantly shifts from you both being lovers to being a couple in love. Sex tips with this change, with lust morphing into romance, torrid kissing getting replaced by intense eye-gazing, greedily devouring each other's bodies with your eyes turning into examining each other's faces. If intimacy increases even further, a fiercely powerful friendship muscles its way into the mix, pushing sexual passion even further out of the equation. Your heart might soar when you hear your partner describe you as their best friend, but it can be the kiss of death for your sex life. Despite films like *My Best Friend's Wedding*, most of us really *don't* want to make love to our friends. It would feel incestuous, like having sex with a sibling, not to mention highly embarrassing.

> 'My wife is the person I tell everything to. If anything happened to her I would lose the person I hold dearest in the world. I find it alarming that I want to have sex with other women, despite feeling like this. I don't act on it, but I find even the tartiest girl far, far more appealing than my wife, even though she's worth a hundred of them. It upsets me.'
>
> James, 43

One of the world's leading experts in the intimacy-versus-sex debate is Jack Morin, author of *The Erotic Mind* – essential reading for any couple struggling with this issue, by the way. Morin and others are at the forefront of exploring why closeness destroys rather than enhances sex (as we've always assumed). The reason appears to be this simple: we find 'separateness' far more attractive. We need to see our partners as individuals, people who are their own person rather than one half of ourselves, in order to fancy them. If you become emotionally fused to the point where you lose your sense of where you finish and they start, you don't just lose your identity, you lose interest. Genuine closeness is a turn-off. Familiarity and comfort are welcome bedfellows for relationships but they're lethal for your love life.

Healthier is what's called 'differentiation': you're emotionally engaged and connected but you accept that you're two separate people who don't have to agree on everything, do everything together or like the same things. You don't merge you *complement* each other. A crucial ingredient to having good long-term sex is novelty: if you've become matching bookends with the same tastes and views, that's hard to achieve. If you think the same, you'll both come up with the same ideas and dismiss ones that don't appeal instantly, knowing your partner won't be attracted either.

Differentiated couples embrace their differences and push each other out of their comfort zones, challenging their partner to try new things and see things from a different point of view.

The other paradox is that the more you value your relationship, the more difficult it is to sustain passion. According to Morin, if you have everything to lose, you're far less likely to take risks – and taking the right kind of risks is crucial to solving the intimacy-versus-sex conundrum. The reason why first-time sex is such a turn-on is because it's unfamiliar to us. Unfamiliarity makes us both anxious and excited, and the resulting euphoria is addictive. Ever had to make a speech where you're nearly throwing up beforehand but have to be dragged away from the microphone once you've been up there for ten minutes? Most people glide off the stage, floating on a cloud of exhilaration. Sadly, there's a limit to how many physical 'firsts' we can have with our partners – first hug, first kiss, first time naked, first oral sex, first intercourse etc – which is why desire fades fast. Familiarity breeds boredom.

Morin believes passion is created when there's the right mix of 'anxiety tolerance' (we're emotionally healthy enough to cope with being stretched) and challenge. In short, we should push ourselves sexually, then when we've mastered that particular thing, aim for something that's just a little further out of our reach. Something we haven't done before is something unknown and unfamiliar. Bingo.

If you think this all sounds suspiciously like I'm going to advise a certain amount of kinky sex, you're probably right. Morin calls an 'eyes-open orgasm' one where we let our partners see our true erotic selves: 'What's really going on inside those murky depths,' he says, somewhat cheerfully. I don't know about you, but there's some pretty kinky stuff in *my* murky depths (so to speak) so I'm presuming there's some in yours as well. Instead of shying away from this side of ourselves, the secret appears to be welcoming it.

Experts now believe the only way to keep passion alive is to have the courage to let your partner see the real sexual you – the naughty one. The not-so-ladylike, politically incorrect you. Sides of you that even *you* find uncomfortable. I'm not pretending it's not *bloody* risky to do this. It is. Which, to go back to my earlier point, is why close, valued relationships are the least likely to encourage it. If your top priority is to be liked by your partner and to minimize the chances of you splitting, this sounds like a recipe for disaster rather than lifelong happiness. It's scary seeing sides to your partner you weren't aware existed. You feel like you don't know them at all. It works wonders for your sex life – it feels risky, edgy, dangerous, all of which make us feel aroused – but it also pushes us unceremoniously out of the warm, comfy marital bed where we knew our partner better than we know ourselves.

Equally, if not more risky, is baring your soul and being seen exactly as you are, rather than the cleaned-up, toned-down version we present. But it's essential, says Morin: having the guts to be yourselves and ask for things knowing you won't be judged is the key to fantastic long-term sex.

So, the answer to the question, 'Are you too close for great sex?' could well be yes. But you're not being asked to ditch intimacy, just to unpeel the Velcro that's attaching you hip-to-hip and stand facing each other, rather than side by side. To take a little tiny step away from each other; to wave each other out the door occasionally.

> 'Sorry, honey, I have a headache' should be 'Yes please, I have a migraine'! A Chicago study shows migraine sufferers want sex more than people with other kinds of headaches. The link between desire and migraines may be because they're both influenced by the same brain chemical, serotonin.

When couples do dare to expand their range of solo interests and become more engaged and stimulated by the outside world, typically their attraction for each other grows, says Morin. 'Insecurity about what your partner is doing might feel uncomfortable but it heightens your interest,' he says. It especially means letting those X-rated, wicked thoughts work their way to the forefront of our brains rather than pushing them back. It means revealing them to our partners and letting them reveal theirs. Acting on some of them, feeling a little out of control, feeling anxious but oddly turned on. Feeling, in fact, like having a jolly good . . . I think you get the picture. One final word: if you're going to do this, do it soon. 'I've never seen a couple who were able to rebuild a sexual connection after they had stopped thinking of each other erotically for five or more years,' Morin warns. How long has it been for you?

YOUR STEAMIEST SEX WISH GRANTED (WITHOUT SCARING HIM OFF IN THE PROCESS)

There's a perception that women are the ones who react with horror if their partner confesses a desire to do dark, dirty deeds, but in reality it's often men who feel most threatened. *You* asking *him* to up the erotic ante means you're reversing the traditional sexual roles, which can be emasculating. 'It's a bit like guys boasting about how they'd love it if a girl came up to them in a bar and said, "Take me home now",' says Robert, a 32-year-old banker friend of mine. 'Most men would run if it actually happened. We're meant to be the sexual predator and instigator of kinky things, not her.'

There's a certain type of man who will react to any suggestion of spicing up your sex life with disapproval. Women – delicate little petals that we are – aren't supposed to want naughty things and this man's judgement of you will be rapid and harsh: you're a tart or a slut and definitely not good enough to be sitting at his parents' table for Sunday lunch. Quite frankly, if you seriously think this is the reaction you'd get from your other half, not being able to share sexual fantasies is the least of your problems and you might want to rethink your choice of partner. It's one thing being tactful and diplomatic about your sexual needs, but quite another having to bury them because you've hooked up with someone who's intent on making you feel bad about yourself. Most of us do a pretty good job of doing that ourselves, thanks very much.

> **❶** *The person who says 'we' the most during an argument, puts forward the best solutions. 'We' users are better at compromising and come up with win-win solutions. 'You' users criticize, disagree, justify and use other negative ploys.*

Happily, despite all the potential pitfalls, there are ways to have your orgasms and keep him too. It's simply a matter of following some simple rules and understanding possible qualms about the particular fantasy you hanker after. But before we get into that, these are the basics which you should apply to any situation where you're suggesting something new sexually:

- **Make it his idea:** Any good negotiator will tell you someone is far more open to doing something if they think the idea came from them. He's always saying he'd love to get his boss back? What better way than to be totally disrespectful and have sex on his desk after hours as long as you don't get caught?

- **Make it clear you've only ever wanted to do it with him:** His first thought will be, Has she already done this with someone else? If you *have* done it with someone else, tell a white lie and give the impression he's just awakened an incredibly erotic side of you.

- **Make it clear you're suggesting it because you trust him:** You know you won't be judged and he's made you feel so good about yourself, you feel you can truly open up and tell him anything.

- **Tell him you're suggesting it because you want to have the best sex life possible:** You know all the statistics about couples cheating on each other and don't want that to happen to you two. You're trying to make sure your sex life stays as exciting as possible so he doesn't feel the need to stray.

- **Be aware that most men feel threatened by the new breed of sexually confident women:** No matter how liberated he is, you have to remember the poor little sausage is just getting over the horrific news that his penis alone often can't give you an orgasm. Most men will enthusiastically welcome exploring your sexual fantasies once their fears are allayed, but it really is crucial for you to present your proposition tenderly and tactfully rather than assume he's up for anything just because he's a man.

OK, now we've got the basics out of the way, read on for specific tips on how to approach a fantasy that does it for you.

Sex with another woman

Most men love it if you admit to indulging in lusty lesbian fantasies, so why not take it through to reality? If your partner's not the jealous type and it's a relatively new relationship you don't mind risking, go right ahead and suggest it. This isn't as straightforward for a long-term partner, though. For some, monogamy is monogamy, regardless of gender, and you're suddenly in a whole lot of trouble for daring to entertain such thoughts. Simply asking to do it counts as infidelity for lots of people and quite a number of men I spoke to said they'd actually prefer their partner indulge without ever telling them. Speaking of which, why are you telling your partner? Are you after his permission, do you want him to join in or watch or are you simply telling him it's something you're going to do? Is this is a one-off experience or something you want to do regularly?
Suggest it by: Thinking all this through before opening your mouth, and when you do, broach the idea by telling him you had an incredibly erotic dream last night about you and another woman in whichever scenario you crave. See what reaction you get. It's pretty easy to move from here it into a serious discussion.

A threesome

To say you need to tread carefully and tactfully when negotiating this one is like reminding you not to turn up with *Bride* magazine when your girlfriend's just been jilted at the altar. Just because he's always joking about it doesn't mean he really wants to try it. It's macho to think he could handle two women or be cool enough to have another man in his bed. Faced with it happening in reality, all sorts of fears creep in.

Suggest it by: Pretending you saw a magazine story about threesomes and how they're becoming more common, then ask, 'What do you think of them?' If he doesn't react with absolute horror, confess you'd like to try it, then talk about the reasons why it appeals, being tactful, tasteful and loading on the sexual compliments. If you decide to go ahead, always, always practise safe sex, never have a threesome unless both of you want one and make rules on what is and isn't allowed re kissing, touching, oral sex, penetration and anal play. Don't take being left out personally, stop if you become upset and always pay your partner more attention than the third person.

Role-play

Acting out a role-play is relatively tame compared to threesomes or swinging but it's still a dreaded scenario for many guys. Why? The risk of humiliation is high because you both have to 'act'. If he's shy, playing the well-hung postman who delivers more than just the mail is living hell, and even if he's not, fears that he'll burst out laughing at the sight of you dressed up as Madonna (offending you for ever) plague him. And that's if you're suggesting something that's not too out of the ordinary.

Suggest it by: Choosing your moment and making a joke of it. Say, 'A girl at work was chatting to me about how she and her boyfriend dress up and act out scenarios. What do you think about that?' His answer may well be 'Silly' or 'I'd laugh', to which you answer, 'I'd probably feel silly and laugh, too, but it might be fun. How about doctors and nurses, didn't you play that as a kid?' Once you've let him know it doesn't have to be deadly serious, the chances are he'll come round to the idea. Stop the giggles if they do happen by fast-forwarding to a particularly raunchy part: sensation should over-ride embarrassment.

Spanking

Spanking puts one of you in the power position, and because hurting others or letting them hurt you is unacceptable, it's an instant aphrodisiac. Some men think it's degrading to spank their partner – and it definitely is if you don't ask for it – but *wanting* them to spank you is quite another thing.

Suggest it by: Visiting a good sex shop or going online and buying a rubber whip – they look fierce but are super-soft – but *only* if you're pretty confident he'll get a buzz from it. Give it to him along with a note detailing what you'd like him to do to you. If you're a little nervous, buy a book with a spanking scene in it and read bits out loud to your partner. His reaction – interest or disgust – will speak volumes.

Keep it light-hearted to start with: use soft whips rather than hard, serious-looking paddles, silk scarves or stockings rather than dangerously real handcuffs. And please, no gimp masks or studded collars until you're both complete converts.

> **Around 50 per cent of women and 75 per cent of men fantasize during sex with a partner. We do it mainly at the beginning to increase arousal and at the end to tip us over into orgasm.**

Having phone sex/talking dirty

'The first time I talked dirty, the guy I was with lost his erection and told me I was a slut. Needless to say, I'm a little nervous suggesting it again even though I love doing it and love it when guys do it to me.' I get letters like this from women all the time and there's a common theme throughout: confusion. Like, he watches porn all the time and swears and carries on with his friends, why wouldn't he like talking dirty? What's going on?

The sort of men who tend to react badly are usually traditional, conservative men, brought up in a household where sex was dirty and good girls definitely didn't. But even 'normal' men sometimes find it difficult to speak 'badly' to their girlfriends or hear very rude things coming out of her mouth. It seems disrespectful, which is, of course, why talking dirty and phone sex work a treat: they make us feel sexually uncomfortable and sometimes that's a good thing.

Suggest it by: Upping your moans and groans, then slipping in the odd swear word or phrase and seeing what he does. If he seems to like it, start describing what's happening: 'I'm watching you disappear inside me and that is *so* sexy.' If you want him to talk dirty to you, follow this by whispering, 'Tell me what you'd *really* like to do to me,' in his ear. If he looks horrified, give a little giggle to lighten it all up. Explain to him that he doesn't have to use swear words or be offensive to be sexy and that he shouldn't worry if he thinks he sounds cheesy or clichéd – nearly all dirty talk is! If you're having phone sex, you've got an advantage – he can't see you, so you can shamelessly nick stuff from erotic books or lads' mags.

Watching (very naughty) porn

Nothing divides opinion quicker than a discussion about pornography: for everyone who considers it a harmless male pursuit or uses it to boost a lacklustre sex life, there's another self-righteous soul who turns puce at the mere mention of a girlie pic or flick and thinks the whole thing is wrong, wrong, *wrong*! And it's not just the grannies kicking up a fuss, I know plenty of young, attractive men and women who have a real problem with porn. Women worry because they don't look or act like female fantasy stars, but often it's him who's threatened by the stars – you envy the breasts, he wants the enormous penis and performance. He may also be shocked by a female appreciating good-quality pornography because . . . well, we're not really supposed to be into dirty sex, are we? This is why suggesting you both watch a XXX-rated film together might not be the walk in the park you think. **Suggest it by:** Bringing home some hot films and watch his reaction. Snuggle up and say 'God, this is hot! Are you enjoying it?' If you get a nod say, 'Maybe we should try watching something even naughtier together. What do you think?' Choose mild stuff for the first few sessions, then inch your way (literally) toward hard core. Don't be alarmed, by the way, if you find yourself enjoying stuff that's not aimed at you. Plenty of women love watching lesbian porn without it making them bisexual or gay, and there's a growing number of straight women who massively enjoy gay male porn. No prizes for guessing why: the men are way better looking than in straight porn and the bodies are to die for!

> 'To me pornography is sexual gluttony. I equate it to over-eating as opposed to having a nice meal in a restaurant, where I've savoured each mouthful and left sated not stuffed. It's an excess of everything. It doesn't appeal to me.'
>
> Tony, 39

SHOW AND TELL FOR GROWN-UPS

The only, absolutely guaranteed way to find out how your partner likes to be brought to orgasm manually is to watch them do it to themselves. Watching your partner masturbate isn't just sexy, it's the most informative sex lesson you'll get. Too embarrassed to demonstrate? Close your eyes as you're doing it. I don't care if you're dying ➤

behind those eyelids, the benefits of doing this far outweigh the angst, so stop being a wimp and get on with it. While you're watching each other, pay special attention to:

HIM:

- **Where he places his hand at the very start:** This is crucial. Adopting the exact position of his hand and fingers is the key to replicating what he does. Ask him to stop the minute he's taken hold of himself and take a good look. Get him to remove his hand and put yours in what you think is the exact same position. Does he agree you've got it right?

- **What pressure, speed and rhythm he uses:** Put your hand over his once he gets going to get a better idea of the speed and rhythm. Once you've got the general idea, let him continue solo.

- **What alters from his first hand motion to orgasm:** Does he maintain the same technique or switch between several? Does he speed up on approach to orgasm? Does he use his free hand to stimulate any other areas like his testes or lower tummy?

- **What happens to his body on approach to orgasm:** You'll probably notice his testes will rise towards his body, his penis will become purplish in colour and his breathing will alter. Also look for his 'orgasm face' – a tell-tale expression that he's about to climax. Is his head thrown back? What noises is he making?

- **When he stops stimulation:** Once you can see he's crossed the line into ejaculatory inevitability – he's about to orgasm no matter what – what happens next? When does he stop moving his hand? Does he remove it completely or hold onto his penis till the very end? How is he holding it?

HER:

- **Where she places her fingers at the very start:**
  Does she use lubricant or saliva to make the area slippery? Does she go straight for the clitoris or touch other areas of her vulva or body first? What position is she in? What does she do with her spare hand? Does she stimulate her breasts?

- **What pressure, speed and rhythm she uses:** It's fine for her to show you how she masturbates using her vibrator, but more helpful if she can repeat the process at some stage using just fingers. Look at the angle of her fingers, what part of the finger she's using, how many, how she's rubbing, how hard and how fast. Does she concentrate purely on her clitoris or alternate between this and inserting a finger/fingers inside? Does there appear to be an order? Put your hand over hers to feel as well as see exactly what's happening. If she's shy, sit behind her and let her lean back against your chest, relaxing between your legs, then put your hand over hers. Don't stay in this position, though, you need to move back in front of her to observe properly. Get her to close her eyes if she finds this threatening.

- **What alters from her first touch through to orgasm:** It's probable she'll stick to the same technique on approach to orgasm, and it's also likely it won't alter much (apart from speed) throughout the whole session. Women tend to like predictability in orgasm, and rather than craving variety with hand masturbation are often happiest if you do exactly the same thing each time. As always, though, just because most women like something doesn't mean all do. Watch to see if she stops and starts or keeps moving her fingers continuously. ➢

- **What are the tell-tale signs she's approaching orgasm:** You'll probably notice her clitoris will become more erect, the colour of her genitals will become redder and brighter, she'll breathe differently and her nipples may harden. Lots of women tip their heads back and lots briefly develop a red rash on their upper chest. What are *her* personal signals?

- **When does she stop stimulation?** This is *crucial* and the most important part of the whole exercise. One of the most common mistakes men make when masturbating a women is stopping too soon. Our orgasms take much longer than yours, so you might be surprised (not to mention jealous) to see she keeps moving her fingers for much longer than you do when you do it to her. Note also the pressure and speed. Does she increase both, then decrease significantly during orgasm? At what point does she withdraw her fingers completely?

DIY SEX THERAPY: THINK LIKE A SHRINK

It takes a couple an average of seven years to seek help with a relationship problem, according to statistics from the John Gottman Institute, yet it's now a matter of weeks before the average person will seek medical advice once a symptom presents itself. Why we'll happily pop off and see an ear, nose and throat specialist when we've got tender tonsils, but won't call a relationship or sex therapist if we've having trouble with our heart or parts is a never-ending source of frustration for me.

I've cheerfully (well, maybe not at the time) seen a psychologist or counsellor at various stages of my life. I went for a session or two when I emerged from a bad relationship to figure out what sent me there in the first place, I went for a number of sessions to help me stop smoking, I went for one 'check-up' when I left my marriage to work out if I'd left for the right reasons – and I'll go again if I strike a period of my life where I feel I need a good, expert, objective opinion. Why can't I fix myself or call on friends who are therapists and sex therapists? Because sometimes I, and they, are too close to the situation to be objective. Other times, I want a viewpoint apart from my own, because my friends and I tend to think alike. It's not admitting failure if you see or would like to see a 'shrink', it's recognizing that an expert is likely to solve the problem twenty-five times faster than you will on your own.

> 'When I was about fifteen I lost my virginity to one of the instructors at school camp. She was three years older than me. The first thing she did after we had sex was make me watch her bring herself to orgasm with her fingers. "This is how most women do it," she said. I've never forgotten it.'
>
> Steve, 28

Having had my rant, I still know lots of you would prefer to be a pedestrian trapped in the middle of a frenetic eight-lane highway at rush hour than lie for five minutes on a couch (most therapists don't make you do that, by the way). So, in an attempt to make sure you don't miss out on the infinite wisdom you might get from a professional, I've compiled a taster of the type of things you might have been told – a combination of core principles, strategies and wise words. I hasten to add, by the way, that these come from the lips of 'active' therapists rather than the clichéd, old-fashioned types who simply sit there, offer nothing and say, 'What do *you* think?' It's meant to work on two levels: to let you see how non-threatening and helpful the process can be if you do choose to go along – and to get you to 'think like a shrink' in case you don't.

Basically, all a therapist does is try to get you to drop those defensive strategies that stop you seeing the truth about yourself and others. Once you've done this, you're able to understand and challenge yourself, your partner and your key issues.

- **Be sensitive to your partner's efforts:** If they greet you at the door stark naked and you walk straight past, throwing a 'What's for dinner?' over your shoulder, they're going to be devastated, not to mention thoroughly and justifiably pissed off. If you're both actively trying to solve a problem, reward every single effort your partner makes, no matter how small (or how hungry you are at the end of the day).

- **How healthy are your intimate relationships generally?** Are you well liked at work? Do you have close friends and get on well with your family? In other words, how do you relate to people? It's useful to know whether your problems are specific to your relationship or something one or both of you struggle with generally.

- **Take a close look at your parents:** Like it or not, how you relate to other people, most particularly your partner, is nearly always based on how you related to your family while growing up. We tend to take on the role of our childhood selves when in a romantic relationship, or turn into one of our parents. This will either make you feel warm and fuzzy (rushing over to kiss the huge photograph you have of your parents above the mantelpiece) or like sticking your head in an oven (your parents' picture doubles as a dartboard). Look at yourselves and each other for astute observations.

- **Compromise isn't always the solution:** Sometimes, meeting in the middle leaves everyone unsatisfied. If it's the *way* you have sex that's causing problems, rather than the frequency, having sex his way one time, and hers the next can just lead to frustration on both parts, with neither of you enjoying the other's turn. Compromise is good, but there are other solutions.

- **It's what you *do* sexually that's important, not what you *think*:** Don't get all hung-up or guilty about any naughty thoughts you have or have had. Fleeting thoughts about what it might be like to sleep with your best friend/partner's worst enemy/the dog don't mean a thing. We are defined by our sexual behaviour not our sexual impulses. Don't try to analyse, explain or justify what appear to be out-of-character flashes of lust. We all have bizarre thoughts. Ever sat in your car, pulled up at a pedestrian crossing, and wondered what would happen if you put your foot on the accelerator and drove straight into the people walking across the road? Does this make you a homicidal maniac who should be locked up? Of course not. (Or maybe I should be locked up. Please tell me everyone's thought that and it's not just me?)

  > '*Blirtatious*' *women, who talk long and freely, initially appear as a Godsend to a shy man. Long term, though, he's less enamoured. As time goes by she talks more and more in an effort to draw him out, giving him less and less time to work up to saying something.*

- **Don't be threatened by your partner, they're the same as you:** They might seem more together/more glamorous/sexier/more confident than you, but we're all the same underneath. We all want to be loved and to feel secure and we all want sexual satisfaction, whatever that means to us. We also tend to crave money, power and other less than altruistic things, like Prada handbags, red sports cars and a bigger, better house than our best friends' have.

- **People often act exactly the opposite of the way they feel:** Shy people, desperately trying to appear cool and in control, come across as arrogant. People who refuse to wear their glasses for vanity reasons appear unfriendly because they can't *see* friends, so fail to acknowledge them. A partner who is desperately worried about losing you is frightened, so lashes out rather than holds you close. Someone who would cut off their right arm to know you really, really do find them attractive after all, will coldly fob off any compliments.

- **Pick your time to talk and use the right language:** Discussions have most impact when you're both in a positive mood and are really keen to fix things, or you're at rock bottom and know you'll split unless you do. I don't think I need to point out the first option is preferable? When it does happen, remember that listening is more important than talking, talk about how you feel rather than how they make you feel – 'I feel upset' rather than 'You make me upset' – ask for what you want more of rather than focus on what you're *not* getting and throw in compliments, whatever you're talking about. An off-hand, 'And my God, while we're on the topic of sex, can I just tell you how *fanbloodytastic* that was last night,' tossed into the middle of a tactful discussion about how you'd like sex more often can sway them to your way of thinking more effectively than an hour of logical reasoning. We like people who make us feel good, so use this to your advantage.

- **Make your point three times, three ways:** This ensures your partner really has understood it. Some people are auditory and like hearing things, others are visual and want to be shown, kinesthetic people are best reached by appealing to their feelings. Use different language or a different means of communication – writing something down, drawing a picture, giving a demonstration – each time you repeat your point and you've got more chance of them understanding.

- **Ageing doesn't destroy sex, attitude does:** When people talk about reaching a sexual peak, they're talking about your genitals. Genitals reach peak responsiveness in adolescence but this simply means that *physically* you're at your peak. An eighteen-year-old recovers rapidly from an orgasm and is physically capable of having another a lot faster than a man in his forties, for instance. But, as US psychiatrist Emanuel H. Rosen says, 'It can take half a century to get your heart and judgement involved. Genital prime and sexual prime are entirely different.' It's often said that women reach their sexual peak in their thirties. This has nothing to do with our physical make-up and everything to do with our attitude to sex. Women tend to be more relaxed about their bodies and know more about what they need to orgasm in their thirties than they do in their teens, plus they have the confidence to tell a lover what they like. Is it any wonder they enjoy sex more? So while our bodies might be physically past their peak, it's entirely possible to reach your sexual prime in your forties, fifties, sixties . . .

- **Be the first to reach out and touch:** It doesn't really matter what you do or even if it's sexual or not, so long as one of you reaches out to break the drought, you're on the way to being 'fixed'. Increase the amount of physical contact you have and you'll nearly always benefit as a couple.

- **Sex is critical no matter what anyone says:** When it's good, it only accounts for around a quarter of your enjoyment of the whole relationship. When it's bad, it can poison the other three-quarters. Don't believe couples who tell you sex is over-rated: it's under-rated, not over-rated. Sex is one of life's greatest pleasures and the most profound way to show how much we love someone. Forget paying off the mortgage in record time. Make that your prime focus at the expense of sex and laughter and you'll end up having to sell the house because one or both of you will have an affair.

THE SEX DETOX:
Would a sex contract work for you?

Lots of sex therapists advise couples to sign 'sex contracts' as an effective, controlled way to get things back on track. They claim that not only does this show serious commitment to the therapy, but without pre-planning, real life tends to take over and very little is accomplished. Organized, systematic people who are used to making to-do lists, usually don't have a problem with a sex contract. People used to operating spontaneously, with a strong dislike of rules, commitment or authority, find the idea repellent.

The fact is, no matter which statistic or study you choose to quote, planning is a central element to success in almost all projects. So there's good reason to push yourself out of your comfort zone, take a deep breath and give it a go. Like most fears, actually doing something – in this case committing sexually to your partner – usually turns out to be far less frightening in reality than the concept of it. If one or both of you still has your nose crinkled in disgust, you can still get a lot out of the sex detox by simply doing the exercises without formulating or signing the contract. Before you completely dismiss the idea, though, here are some reasons why you might want to reconsider:

Why a contract works:
- Commitment to the contract is commitment to each other.
- Because you have to write things down, it forces you to think in specifics.
- Also because it's written, it makes things real. You can't escape from your promises to each other because they're in front of you in black and white.

- It keeps you focused. It's incredibly easy to get waylaid and go off track when you're trying to change behaviour. It's far simpler to tread a familiar path than go somewhere new, the trouble is the known road takes you back to where you were at the start. If that happens, couples usually decide the whole exercise has been pointless because they've failed. In reality, the plan didn't fail, you just didn't make yourselves stick to it until it became second nature.
- Having a plan that spells out your problems, needs and wants as well as solutions is reassuring for lots of couples.
- You can chart your progress, giving you an incentive to keep going.
- Sex contracts often morph into simple lists of what each of you would love to try or enjoyed immensely. These can continue indefinitely.

The detox

This programme is based on fairly standard advice from respected sex therapists. If you like the sound of it and want more detail, I highly recommend *Electrify Your Sex Life* by Carole Altman. This detox is deliberately non-specific to provide you with a framework which you can personalize. There isn't the space to include a complete plan, but I've included sample exercises. You'll notice – shock horror! – I've suggested you abstain from all sexual contact for three weeks. There's a reason for each week I'm making you go without it: first, it makes you focus on non-sexual interaction and gives you a clear view of your sex life. Second, sex during this period, while you're intensely dissecting everything, can feel rather self-conscious. Finally, stopping sex, then reintroducing it a little at a time, is what detoxes you. It takes you both back to basics, forces you to concentrate and in doing so helps break bad habits.

Contract one

I agree not to have sex at all for one week so we can focus fully on examining our sex life, isolating any problems and working on solutions. Neither of us will initiate sexual contact, other than affectionate kissing or hugging, and neither of us will feel guilty for not having sex or feel pressured to have it.

What to do

- To get a broad idea of what you both think about sex in general, write down anything and everything you think about your sex life. Here are some questions you might ponder, but don't just write yes or no answers, include at least one or two sentences to explain why:

- Do you enjoy sex?
- Do you masturbate?
- What part of sex do you like the most?
- Do you think you know your partner's sexual needs and wants?
- How do you know? What led you to these conclusions?
- Do they know yours?
- What signals have you given your partner to give a clear idea of your needs and wants?
- Is there something you'd like to try but are too afraid to ask?
- What do you think will happen if you suggest it?
- How would you rate your sex life on a scale of one to ten?
- What needs to happen to make that score higher?
- Are you happy about your body?
- Is there anything sexual you absolutely wouldn't do?
- What do you most want to change about your sex life?
- What do you want to stay the same?

When you've done your lists separately, swap and discuss what you've come up with. Don't worry if you feel a bit prickly, any criticism is hard to take initially. Remember you're working as a team to make your sex life better, rather than pointing fingers. It's never one person's fault, it's how the two of you are inter-relating.

- The next session, move on to ways to improve your sex life. Write down the twenty things you most like about what your partner does, then ten things you would like more of and why, giving at least two sentences of specific details. For instance, 'I'd like you to kiss my neck more often because that's a hot spot for me. Can you do it hard, to the point where you're almost biting me? I'd especially like it if you do this during intercourse when I'm about to orgasm.'

  You'll both feel like twits when you start writing stuff like this down, but once you get started it's incredibly liberating. Be tactful and sensitive but be truthful. So long as you concentrate on what you want more of, rather than what your partner's doing wrong, you're unlikely to offend.

- Work out when you'll both have time to try out the techniques and 'homework' for the next two-week contract. Naming days and specific times is better than just allotting a lump of time.

Contract two

I agree to spend the next two weeks focusing on our sex life so we can explore new ways to make it even better. I agree not to have sex and instead enjoy non-sexual touching, cuddling and kissing. The time I intend to devote to this is (name specific times and days) and nothing but an emergency will stop me honouring this promise.

What to do

- Try some intimacy exercises: these are simply things that bring you closer. Carole Altman suggests you both sit opposite each other, legs crossed on the bed, and stare into each other's eyes and faces for a full five minutes (use a timer). Really look at your partner and see them as they are. Yes, you'll giggle, but just keep going. We all have an image of our partner which we carry around in our heads and often it's based on when we first met. The person before you has changed since then. Notice the changes with a positive slant, i.e. how much wiser they look, rather than, *Jesus!*, when did they start looking this old? Then take each other's hands and examine those for a further five minutes. For the next step, remove your clothes and examine each other's bodies – five minutes again – but *only* using your hands and eyes. Remember, you're exploring and observing *not* stimulating. Even if you do find this as sexy as hell, don't act on it or deliberately touch to turn on. Don't speak during the exercise. Once you've finished, give each other a rundown on what felt good, what didn't and what you discovered about each other. Take turns talking, again using the timer. Each gets to speak for five minutes.
- Other exercises during this period could include stress-reduction/relaxation exercises, imagery exercises to encourage you both to fantasize and exercises to improve your communication. The Sensate Focus Program (covered briefly on page 206) is also popular.

Contract three

I agree to one week of sexual contact but without penetration of any type. Instead, I will explore other methods to make both of us orgasm. The time I intend to devote to this is (name specific times and days) and nothing but an emergency will stop me honouring this promise.

What to do

- Take your pick from any of the techniques in this book that don't involve intercourse or penetration and give them a whirl. No penetration, by the way, means no penis, fingers or sex toys inserted into vaginas or bottoms.
- Have a shower or bath together, soaping each other and observing what your partner likes and doesn't like. At this point, it's OK to give a running commentary as it happens, rather than waiting until afterwards because you both should now be in the habit of talking freely and spontaneously about your feelings and sensations. Move from the shower or bath to the bed for good old-fashioned body massages, using a variety of touches.
- Flick through this book and each choose two manual masturbation – hands and fingers – techniques you haven't tried and experiment on each other (see pages 98–104) and discuss what you liked or didn't like afterwards. Do the same with two oral sex techniques (see pages 77–87), and again discuss. Try some erotica or sex toys – anything goes at this point except techniques involving penetration.

Contract four

I agree to full sex over the next two weeks, but only under the following circumstances. (Insert what you've learned so far, for example: *If I don't climax through intercourse, I would like you to use your fingers or tongue to make me orgasm either before or after intercourse.*) *I would prefer it if we started off by having sex in this position* (name current favourite positions) *and I'm most likely to feel like it* (insert time of day). *My ideal number of sex sessions over the next two weeks which include intercourse is* (insert number of sessions). *My ideal number of sex sessions which don't include intercourse is* (insert number of sessions). *The time I intend to devote to this is* (name specific times and days) *and nothing but an emergency will stop me honouring this promise. In return I promise to* (list specific things you now know your partner loves. List as many of the things you know they enjoyed, along with how many sessions they have to look forward to of each).

What to do

- Plan your first intercourse encounter enthusiastically. Work out when, where, how and what you can do to make it even more special. It'll be special, believe me (you haven't had intercourse for four weeks!)
- Choose five new intercourse positions each (see pages 52–6 for inspiration) and try two each future session.
- Simply put into practice everything in the contract for the next two weeks.

It's usually at this point that couples start to realize just how much effort they're now putting into their sex life, and how little they did before. It's also around now that you start to realize spontaneity was sacrificed for this six-week period for good reason. Not only should you both know infinitely more about each other's emotional needs, you should have a very clear idea of where, how and why your partner likes to be touched, specifically what they'd be up for in the future – and know they know the same about you. Add to that a host of new positions and techniques you've added to your repertoire and you can see why some couples continue to make contracts, even if most tend to end up as simple lists of what they'd next like to try and when.

It takes six weeks to make a change permanent so both continue to make a concentrated effort to put all you've learned into practice during this time. After that, it should become part of your natural behaviour.

THE TECHNIQUES SEX THERAPISTS REALLY RATE

Sex therapists are obviously individuals with their own favourite tried-and-tested methods, but there are some fairly standard procedures followed for common problems. If you want to practise effective DIY sex therapy at home this will give you an idea of how to do it and also provide insight on what would happen if you did seek professional help.

The basic steps:
As a general guide to solving problems, it's recommended you do the following:

- **Acknowledge something is wrong and identify the symptoms** – here's the hard part – **without blaming anyone**. This requires both good communication and good grace.
- **Check out possible medical causes** by visiting your GP for a full check-up. And yes it does mean telling the truth about your lifestyle, including 'fessing up to any recreational drug use, excessive drinking or embarrassing prescription medications for things like irritable bowel syndrome or anti-depressants – especially anti-depressants, which are a known libido slayer.
- **Educate yourselves:** Start by looking up a good, modern sex reference book, then find more specialized titles. Or go online and search for support groups and/or information or websites which appear to be medical or scientifically based or affiliated with an organization or individual who appears trustworthy.
- **Try not to be biased in your diagnosis** of what needs to be done to fix the problem. Men prefer things to fit nicely under the medical heading because it means it's not their fault and it's a lot less scary than having to do all that talking and exploring of emotions. The truth is, sex problems nearly always involve mind and body.
- **Try the standard 'cures'** suggested through your research, giving them a good few weeks to begin to make a difference. A good period to allow is six weeks to three months.

- **Seek professional help** if the above don't help the situation, make it worse or you think you'd like professional guidance from the start (see 'Useful Contacts' on pages 288–91).

Common treatments for common problems:

For specific problems, these techniques get good results:

Loss of desire: First, get a referral from your GP to get a full medical to look at what effect lifestyle, general health, medication and your hormone levels are having. If you have private health insurance you can usually claim for a full medical each year though you'll have to ask for hormone level checks to be done on top of this. Some GPs will bill the cost to NHS, others won't. If you get the all-clear, it's worth contacting Relate or BASRT to see a sex therapist (see 'Useful Contacts' on pages 288–91). Fees are based on a sliding scale depending on income. Now you'll be encouraged to look at your relationship in general, and depending on the results, you might be given a testosterone booster (if you're a man, you *must* get your prostate checked first), advised to change contraceptive pills (triphasic pills appear to boost desire) and encouraged to explore your fantasies and/or keep a sex diary. Most sex therapists will also recommend the **Sensate Focus Programme**. This basically involves banning sex and reawakening your sexual feelings by using massage to explore your own, then your partner's body. You first touch yourself all over, taking note of what feels good and arouses you, then you massage each other, avoiding the sex organs, and giving feedback on what feels good. In the final stage, you're allowed to touch the good bits, but only if you give a running commentary of what you're enjoying and what you're not. Finally, you're allowed to have intercourse. (Also see 'Are You Too Close for Great Sex' on page 178 and 'If Sex is So Great, How Come We Don't Have It Any More? on page 212.)

Mismatched libidos: This is a common problem and I've covered it extensively on pages 213–8.

Wanting to be unfaithful: It's not often a person on the brink of an affair will have the sense to turn up at a sex therapist's office asking for help (having done a quick phone around, let me amend 'not often' to 'never') but infidelity is a strong temptation for couples suffering any sort of sexual problem because we all like to kid ourselves it's them, not us, so swapping partners seems like an easy solution. Wanting to have sex with others is something sensation seekers – high-achievers who need a high level of excitement to stay interested – often struggle with, and boredom is a by-product of even the happiest monogamous relationship. Treatments for this include reassurance (there is no such thing as intellectual or emotional fidelity – we *all* fancy other people at some point), fantasy exercises (learning to satisfy the urge by being unfaithful in your head, rather than reality) and generally hotting things up by planning new, edgy erotic adventures.

Impotence: Erectile dysfunction (ED) is not being able to get or maintain an erection sufficiently for intercourse. **Global ED** is not being able to get an erection at all, under any circumstances, and **Situational ED** is not being able to get one with a partner. Don't confuse impotence with low desire. If sex hasn't been great for a while, the chances are your erections aren't as hard as they used to be. It's common in this situation for men to subconsciously 'close' themselves to sex, which can lead to impotence. Other men find they can get an erection without any problems, but it goes down the minute they penetrate. Performance anxiety is often the cause of this type of ED, or (sorry girls) an untoned vagina. As a sex therapist friend of mine says, 'A hand is much firmer than a middle-aged vagina.' Having sex late at night with a belly full of food and alcohol can also affect erections; sex in the morning nearly always produces a harder penis.

The first step if you have ED (the most common) is to check if you get an early-morning erection or can achieve one with masturbation. If you can't, see your GP for a full check-up and ask for a referral to a urologist. If you're able to get erections, it's likely your ED *isn't* caused by physical problems, though an unhealthy lifestyle – too many cigs, alcohol and certain medications – can have an affect. Tackle it by challenging psychological issues, which are often the cause of temporary impotence. This could be as simple as deciding to stop worrying about it. Start having sex without penetration and try *not* to get an erection. If it does happen, ignore it initially – even if you both feel like cracking open champagne – until it's a common occurrence. Once it is, experiment with *brief* penetration by getting her to climb on top, then lift herself off after one or two thrusts before attempting full intercourse. It's usual to try these non-drug methods before succumbing to the little blue Viagra pill or vacuum pumps (see pages 135–7 for details on both).

Retarded ejaculation: This means you're not able to ejaculate when you want to, despite intense and prolonged thrusting or oral sex. 'A problem?' I can hear you say, 'Isn't that a dream come true?' Well, no. It sounds like something you'd boast about down the pub, but if you're a sufferer, you'll know it's frustrating and often painful. It also, ironically, has the opposite effect on women to what you'd expect, causing distress rather than pleasure. She tends to assume it's her fault for not being sexy enough, and he, secretly or not so secretly, sometimes agrees with her because it then means there's nothing wrong with *him*. If you're on anti-depressants, you could already have found the culprit for your tardy orgasms. If it's just started happening and you're tired or under lots of pressure, ditto. Age also has an effect on how quickly you ejaculate, and the amount, by the way. As a young man, you ejaculated roughly a whole teaspoon full. As an older man, that drops to half a teaspoon.

The first step, as usual, is to get a full medical. Prostate problems are sometimes responsible so you must get that checked. Another obvious question to ask is whether you can masturbate yourself to orgasm? If you can, it's probably not a problem that's medically based. Other possible causes include focusing too much on her pleasure, fear of letting go (perhaps because of a previous pregnancy scare or infidelity), or control or power issues in the relationship (you're angry and feel a need to 'withhold').

> **Men fall in love earlier than women and fall out of love later – they're first in, last out. Women are last in, first out – falling in love later and falling out of love sooner.**

Other times it's because you need something to tip you over into orgasm – a finger inserted in the anus, for example – but are too embarrassed to ask your partner to indulge you (will she think I'm gay?).

Desensitization techniques are effective to get you used to ejaculating with a partner rather than just solo. You start by masturbating in a room while your partner is in another room, but with the door open. Then move onto masturbating to orgasm with her standing at the opposite side of the same room, facing away. Work your way closer and closer until you're able to bring yourself to orgasm while she lies beside you. From there on, it's baby steps till you're inside, happily thrusting away, problem sorted.

Premature ejaculation: PE is when a man orgasms too quickly for his, or his partner's satisfaction. As you can appreciate, this might mean anything from five thrusts to fifteen minutes, depending on the people involved. Around 30 per cent of men experience PE at some point, with lots of men ejaculating within two minutes of penetration. Causes include lessons learned from early masturbation (having to get it over with quickly), performance anxiety, not enough regular sex and youth (the younger you are, the more likely it is to happen). The **squeeze technique** is the old, traditional method of dealing with PE. When you're highly aroused, she firmly squeezes the head of the penis for fifteen to twenty seconds, her thumb on the frenulum (the stringy piece of skin where the head connects to the shaft), first and second fingers on the top of the head. Newer, and I think more effective, is the **stop-start technique**. There are several versions of this, but a simple form includes the following steps. **Step one:** You masturbate yourself, getting used to how you feel just before you ejaculate and stopping stimulation before you orgasm. Bring yourself to the brink and stop four times before finally allowing yourself to orgasm and continue this 'training' for several weeks until you feel you know the point you can bring yourself to without letting go. **Step two:** This time she masturbates you, with you telling her when to start and stop. **Step three:** You repeat the initial exercise but inside her. Again, allow yourself to get excited, then stop, then start again. After three or four times peaking, you're allowed to orgasm. The secret to getting the stop-start right is to focus on pleasure and sensation rather than trying to stop yourself ejaculating.

'We went to see a sex therapist and she taught us the stop-start technique to control my partner's premature ejaculation problem. I'd struggled for years to make him visit a professional but he refused. She solved the problem in about a month – something he'd been humiliated by all of his life. He regrets not going sooner.'

Helen, 36

Another simple solution to help PE is for her to take charge during penetration via a woman-on-top position, keeping a close eye on how aroused you're becoming. A further exercise involves learning how to rate your arousal (this is explained on pages 114–15).

Orgasmic difficulties for her: If you're **preorgasmic** you've never had an orgasm, if you're **anorgasmic** you're able to orgasm through masturbation but not able to have one with your partner. Again, get a medical check-up and list any medication you're taking. Other reasons include ineffective sexual technique by your partner, having sexual hang-ups, feeling guilty about sex or thinking it's bad or dirty, not wanting to let go in front of your partner and myriad other reasons.

If you're preorgasmic, the first thing to do is experiment with a vibrator. Almost all women can orgasm this way and you'll then have an idea of what you're aiming for. It's then a matter of training yourself to masturbate with your fingers and being able to share all this with your partner, as well as starting to experiment with oral sex. The Sensate Focus Programme is also recommended.

If you're having problems orgasming with a partner, start focusing on communication: have you told him what turns you on or are you expecting him to be a mind-reader? Is he interpreting your instructions properly? Is he taking time or putting you under pressure? If you're keen to orgasm via penetration, try the 'bridge technique' (page 116) or Coital Alignment Technique (CAT). CAT is an alternative way to have intercourse which involves grinding and rocking rather than in-out thrusting. (My book *Hot Sex* covers this in detail, if you're interested.)

Painful intercourse or vaginismus: In its simplest form, the pain is caused by lack of lubrication – affected by medication, time of month, not enough foreplay, menopause or age – and is fixed by using personal lubricant and spending more time on arousal. But there are lots of other physical reasons ranging from ovarian cysts and infections to Pelvic Inflammatory Disease.

A visit to a gynaecologist is essential. Other things to do are up the amount of foreplay, use lubricant and do Kegel exercises so you feel in control of your vaginal muscles. Vaginismus occurs when the muscles surrounding the vagina contract so tightly that penetration is impossible. Get a medical check-up, see a gynaocologist, then if all seems normal, I'd seriously think about seeing a sex therapist. It tends to be linked to a painful past sexual experience or deeply ingrained attitudes to sex. Not surprisingly, it's common after abuse or rape – in one study, 94 per cent of women who were sexually abused as children had some sexual dysfunction. Being brought up to think sex is bad also tends to feature. The Sensate Focus Programme is recommended, as well as the use of dilators. You start with the smallest dilator, a smooth, hard, cylindrical object, and work up to penis size, inserting it and consciously squeezing and relaxing your PC muscle at the same time. Along with good counselling and an understanding partner, they work well to overcome the PC spasm reflex.

IF SEX IS SO GREAT, HOW COME WE DON'T HAVE IT ANY MORE?

Good point! Why aren't you having it? People who have regular sex are nicer to be around. Sorry for stating the obvious, but there you are. Couples who have regular sex are more happily married than those who don't. I know, one *startling* observation after another. Here's another one: couples who have regular sex are less likely to be tempted by affairs and less likely to divorce. The reason I'm talking to you both like you're ten-year-olds (and dim ones at that) is because I'm trying to explain this the most direct way I can: if you don't have sex any more, you will probably split up.

Assuming you're not ninety-five with a priest hovering by the bed about to deliver the last rites, you are risking your relationship by letting this situation continue. Unless you have a good reason to put sex on the backburner – and there are some (babies, stress, new job, death in the family etc.) – you need to take this seriously.

One of the main reasons couples don't have sex is mismatched libidos. One wants sex lots, the other wants sex less often and the problem becomes so big and fraught with tension you stop having sex completely. This is what I'm going to focus on here: balancing the sexual scales. The trick, of course, is coming up with a compromise, a way to make the highly sexed person feel indulged without the one with a lower libido feeling like they're being taken advantage of. It means thinking outside the box. Sex gets redefined. Having sex together might mean one of you masturbating in front of the other while they look on encouragingly. The horny person is happy and it takes very little effort from the passive partner. The result? Two satisfied customers.

You'll also need a basic understanding of the human response system. Influential author and sex therapist David Schnarch talks about the Quantum Model for sex. It's based on a simple theory that no one single event determines how things will turn out, it's when a lot of different factors all reach a certain level that things happen. Desire is influenced by so many things: our health; what's happening to us at that moment (your partner is stimulating you versus pushing a

> 'Even at the start I always felt like I was coercing my husband into sex. I'd straddle him as we talked and drank and smoked cigarettes, but he seemed much keener on talking than he did on kissing. I pretended to myself that it would get better but it never did. I had an affair, then left.'
>
> Becky, 34

trolley round the supermarket); the intimacy level in your relationship; how much you trust each other; your genes and natural libido level; what you find erotic and how you use it to turn you on; whether you need love to enjoy sex or find it easier to enjoy sex without love. All these factors have to fit together simultaneously to put you in the mood. Then, on top of all that, the male/female arousal systems differ markedly. Think about it. Men can *see* their arousal in the form of a proud, protruding erection and this, in turn, makes them more aroused. Given the female arousal equivalent – lubrication – is happening *inside*, women would want to be in a pretty ambitious lotus position with the neck of a giraffe in order to see theirs.

Schnarch says women are more responsively sexual than spontaneously sexual. He'll walk up to the newsagent, charged with the onerous task of buying a pint of milk, and come back dying for a bit simply because he caught a glimpse of a pouting blonde on the cover of a lads' mag. Women aren't quite as simple (Really? What a shock!). We add other dimensions. Not just, 'but it's 9 a.m. and I haven't had my coffee yet', but, 'do I like my partner today?', 'does he deserve this?', 'what are the kids up to' and 'how tired am I?' If you're a guy and you want sex at 10 p.m., you ought to be behaving yourself and planning it twenty-four hours in advance. Tempted to give up before you've even started? Although this might sound ominous, it's not. Read it through once more and you'll see it's simply a matter of absorbing a few basic principles. Once you've done that, here's some more specific tips for each of you:

A twelve-year study found unhappily married people would be much better off splitting up for general health and happiness levels.

If you've got the higher sex drive

- Masturbate more, hassle your partner less.
- Be acutely aware of what you're craving when you want sex. Men tend to make sexual advances when what they really want is a cuddle. Learn to identify the difference between craving sex or craving affection or security. Women sometimes crave excessive amounts of sex through insecurity. The reasoning being that if he's tuckered out from doing it with you, he's going to be less inclined to chat up the girl with the big knockers down at the pub.
- Be direct when asking for sex and focus on separating sexual and non-sexual affection so there aren't any mixed signals. Discuss and demonstrate the difference between an advance and a romantic gesture. Unzipping your trousers, taking out your penis and saying, 'How can you resist?' counts as an advance.
- Consider formulating a sex contract which spells out an agreed amount of time the two of you will have sex, as well as who initiates it (see pages 198–204). As the high-desire person, you're not allowed to ask for sex at any other time. Oh all right then, it's allowed on your birthday as well.
- Do you know exactly what your partner likes? The better the sex is, the more you'll both want it. Do the 'Show and Tell for Grown-ups' exercise on pages 189–92, and give Chapters 3 and 4 a flick through for tips on technique. Your partner's low desire could be low satisfaction from inept technique. Sorry, but someone has to say it.
- Accept that it's possible for your partner to truly love you and still not want to always have sex with you.
- Don't expect spontaneous desire, accept you may need to create it. Body responsiveness differs from person to person. Some people – you, for instance – need a slightly wicked look sent your way and you're raring to go. Others – your partner – may need lots of kissing, stroking and

general seducing before being persuaded that sex is a good idea. Do whatever it takes to get them in the mood.

- Come up with sexual treats to jolt their desire out of its naturally low setting, such as vibrators, erotica, fantasy, role-play. Help them tap into their naughty side and you'll raise their desire levels.
- Shift the focus during sex to concentrating on stimulating your partner rather than satisfying yourself.
- If sex isn't on the menu, avoid activities which you know turn you on. This means turning off *The Top 100 X-Rated Films* and snuggling up with a copy of *Making Tax Returns Fun*.
- Do more exercise. Feeling edgy, frustrated and slightly furious with your partner for not wanting to get naked? Pull on your running shorts and pound the pavement or hit the gym. It gets rid of excess energy and anger – and if you've joined the *right* gym, you can simultaneously drift into delicious fantasies about the guy/girl running next to you.

If you've got the lower sex drive:

- Just do it. The Nike approach is based on new research which found that for some people sexual desire doesn't come *before* arousal, it comes *after*. If you don't feel in the mood but start having sex, you might then feel aroused enough to continue.
- Desire is a decision. It doesn't just happen, you have to make it happen. Accept responsibility for your arousal, work out what turns you on and do it. Spontaneous lust happens easily in the beginning, but not so easily later on. Sigh wistfully at early memories of the two of you going for it in broom cupboards, but don't think you've failed or don't fancy your partner if you're not panting and shouting 'Yes, honey *now*!' every time they grab your bottom.

- Make a weekly date for sex (minimum) and three other dates (an hour each time) to spend time together outside the bedroom. These dates are *top* of your priority list, not bottom. Putting it after 'organize books into appropriate genre' won't be appreciated. Also consider formulating a sex contract which spells out an agreed amount of time the two of you will have sex, as well as who initiates it (see page 198). When the time comes, *enthusiastically* participate and you might find you enjoy it as much as they do.
- If you're too tired for sex at night, have it in the mornings or afternoons. It's a simple concept, but the simple solutions are often the ones people miss.
- Don't blame. Your partner's not bordering on sex addiction or 'should really see someone' because they want to get horizontal with you. It's a compliment. Fight the 'Why should I do something I don't want to do' indignance and try everything in your power to make sex a pleasure, not a chore.
- Don't wait for a big surge of desire, watch for little flickers. We all feel desire at different levels. If you keep waiting for the moment where you'd cheerfully cut off your limbs to get a bit, you might be waiting an awfully long time. Like seventy years.
- Work out what gets you in the mood and give clear, specific instructions to your partner. If you need time to unwind on your own, tell them. (It's OK to request an hour-long, deep-tissue full-body massage now and then, but making it a 'must do or no can do' is just a teensy bit selfish, don't you think?)
- Work out the effect masturbation has on your sex drive. Some people want sex less if they masturbate regularly, others want it more because their body starts to get used to and crave regular orgasms.
- Have lots of quickies. Everyone can find five minutes in a

day and having lots of quick sex sessions can have a rather interesting effect on your sex life. If five minutes a couple of times a week is all it takes to put a smile on your partner's face while you notice your sex drive is magically boosted, isn't it worth a try?

- Say no without guilt, say yes and give it your all. That, in a nutshell, is the true secret to success. That and saying yes more than once a year.
- How happy are you generally? The better time you're having out of bed, the more likely you are to want to jump in it.
- Read erotica. Let yourself fantasize about whatever the hell you want to. Yes, even small mountain goats.
- Buy a vibrator. Use it solo and during sex with your partner. If you're female, you're far more likely to orgasm during sex, giving you more incentive to want to do it.

7 Same-sex Stuff

The latest on gay, lesbian and bi sex – with tons of tips for straights as well

● ●

There I was in my favourite New York hair salon for the first time in six months, enthusiastically catching up on all the news with the girls on reception. One patted her pregnant tummy, another flashed an engagement ring and Rebecca, the girl who'd had the most chequered, calamitous love life of all, looked simultaneously smug and terrified. I lifted an eyebrow and leaned over to ask conspiratorily, 'So 'fess up, what are *you* up to?'

Rebecca smiled and said, 'Oh I'm really happy.' Nothing else offered.

'So are you in a relationship?' I prodded nosily.

'Um, yes,' she answered.

'Brilliant,' I enthused, 'so who is he and how did you meet?'

Silence. Then a little jerk of her head towards a girl sitting next to her at the counter who I hadn't met before.

'Oh I see,' I said, dropping my voice to a whisper. 'Sorry, I didn't realize you didn't want anyone to know.'

'It's not that,' interjected the girl in a deep, not unattractive masculine voice, 'She means it's *me* she's going out with.'

And they both beamed at me, Rebecca looking remarkably chilled, as if she'd just spent the last six months sunning herself in the Caribbean being hand-fed peeled grapes – (maybe she had?).

Well, bugger me, I thought. 'Well, how about that,' I said. Later, I asked Rebecca if she'd always been gay and just recently had the courage to come out. 'Never fancied another woman in my life,' she said. 'It's not about being gay. It's about meeting one particular person who I adored so much, I didn't care what sex they were.' Now that's what I call being open-minded and not allowing yourself to be put in a box or bound by stereotypes.

That was four years ago and since then I've heard Rebecca's sentiments echoed by other straight/lesbian couples, even two formerly straight girls. Most people's reaction to their unorthodox choice? 'Close girlfriends are a bit taken aback, but then they're cool about it and ask lots of questions. Women generally are intrigued. Men seem slightly uncomfortable at first but soon revert to the clichéd "Can I come and watch?" thing,' says Katie, another person in the same situation.

These days, women sleeping with women really isn't such a big deal. Almost all of the straight women I know have had lesbian snogs, furtive feels, one-nighters or full-on flings at some point in their lives. It's becoming *so* commonplace it's got a lot of people horribly confused. 'Dear Tracey,' wrote one bewildered, elderly gent to my website. 'Is it just me or are lots of women sleeping with other women these days? Was it always like that and I just never noticed?' Bless him. I don't think it was always like that but I do think it's nothing his grandson should be

> **Between 2 and 2.5 per cent of US men are gay and between 1 and 1.4 per cent of US women are lesbian.**

stressing about. Most of the women I know thoroughly enjoyed the experience but have remained straight.

What's interesting is that while gay male couples are certainly more accepted now than they have ever been, straight men wanting to experiment with other men is still taboo. 'If a woman dabbles, she's just dabbling. If a man does it, it means he's secretly gay,' said one of the people I interviewed – and he was gay, by the way. Lots of people think like this. Two women together seem to be a turn-on to almost everyone – straight guys, straight girls, gay women – whereas two men tends only to put a twinkle in the eye of gay men, though there are women who enjoy male porn simply because the men are more attractive.

> **When one spouse comes out of the closet, a third of couples break up right away while another third stay together for two or three years and then separate. Half of the final third, who opt to try to make it work long-term, split after three years.**

The reason why? While most straight women aren't revolted by the suggestion of sleeping with the same sex, even if it's something which doesn't truly appeal, lots of men are. There's still such a stigma about being a gay man that owning up to even a second-long semi-sexy thought involving another man is frightening. Being gay can lose you friends, jobs, the love of your family and respect of your community. Coming out for men is a *big* decision. So is it any wonder they don't allow themselves to even think about straying into that area?

There are all sorts of clichés that apply. Ask most straight people to picture lesbian sex and they'll conjure up nice, soft bodies licking and gently caressing. Ask people to picture two men having sex and it morphs into a rather unsavoury version of a *Carry On* film. One man is usually vigorously pumping his penis into the bottom of another, both men are hairy and sport five o'clock shadows and one is saying, 'Who's your daddy,' in a gruff voice. Imitating a homosexual in a joke, most people adopt queeny, feminine gestures. When it comes to the sex part, there's nothing dainty happening in our imaginations at all.

While nearly all the women I interviewed for this book had a sparkle in their eye when asked if they fancied experimenting with women, only one of the straight men dared even look interested in doing the same with men. He begrudgingly admitted to kissing 'some bloke' once while 'very, very pissed' and feeling 'vaguely interested' in taking it further. Not that he did, *of course*. Highly unfair, yes, but as far as society is concerned, a woman can still be feminine and want to stick her tongue into another woman's whatnot. But a man cannot be seen as manly if he wants to stick *his* bit into another man's anything. Even I, a person who prides myself on being nonjudgemental and rather worryingly aroused by most things (does anyone else see anything sexual about a handsome waiter plunging a spoon of cream deep into the centre of a soufflé?) am not turned on by the thought of a boyfriend secretly panting at the thought of a man-on-man encounter.

A man with older brothers is more likely to be gay because the mother 'fights back' and 'feminises' the foetus. Experts say it's because she's increasingly sensitive to androgen in the womb. This doesn't hold true for women – a girl with many older sisters is not more likely to be gay.

BISEXUAL OR TOO SCARED TO COME OUT?

If you're a female, the answer is probably yes, you are bisexual. If you're a man, it's probably the latter. At least that's the latest view of experts studying the subject. Evidence mounts for a growing case that women are far more 'erotically plastic' than men appear to be. Our sexuality appears to alter depending on our social conditions and environment – we're sexual chameleons. This is why it's entirely possible for us to make an intellectual choice to be a lesbian, rather than feel compelled to do it. The switch works in reverse as well. 'Hasbians', like Anne Heche, were gay but are now heterosexual.

The reason why we're so much more adaptable than men is that we're aroused by more than just what we see. Personality, loyalty, intelligence and kindness are also taken into account and we look at potential partners as people, rather than men. This makes us more likely to fall for the person, rather than the gender. Mother Nature's done it for a reason, of course. Women have to breast-feed both male and female babies, so we need to be open to both sexes getting physically close.

Bisexuality in men, on the other hand, isn't useful for procreation which is why bisexuals and gays form such a tiny percentage of the population. This conclusion was reached by researchers who wired both men and women up to machines that measured blood flow to the sexual organs (a sign of arousal). They were then individually shown a variety of erotic films involving same sex, straight sex and some with primates fornicating. The men in the studies only became aroused when watching men having sex with women or women having sex with each other: the female was the focus. Putting paid to the theory that ➢

So where does all this leave us? Well, a lot more advanced in our attitudes to women, but still hung up on men. I've always found most prejudices are 'cured' when a person is educated about the subject. Hence, this chapter is devoted to same-sex relationships. It's as much aimed at straight people as it is at people already settled with the same sex because a lot of the stuff gays and lesbians get up to straight couples also do, or wouldn't mind having a bash at. Strap-on dildos, learning great hand-job techniques – there's something here for everyone, boys and girls. Even (ouch!) fisting for first-timers. But if anyone shows my mother that bit I'll have to kill them.

Since everyone seems to be doing it or thinking about it, there's also an informative how-to guide for straight girls wanting to sleep with gay girls. And even though it's not quite so popular, a guide for men who fancy a spot of man-on-man action as well. Whatever your sexual orientation, I hope it's all helpful.

IS THERE REALLY SUCH A THING AS A 'GAYDAR'

According to recent research, yes. And guess who's most likely to have a finely tuned one? That's right, other gay men and women. Researchers photographed gay and straight men and women in the same style black top, no jewellery or makeup and from the waist up, and got another group of gay and straight men and women to look at the photos. It took a mere two seconds, literally, for gay men and women to work out who was gay and who wasn't. Straight men – are we surprised? – didn't really have a clue. Interestingly, gay men were easier to recognize than lesbians.

In another experiment which will make you go 'Ewww!' researchers got gay men to sniff T-shirts which had already been worn by gay and straight men. In almost all cases, the gay men preferred the scent of other gay men, while straight women, straight men and lesbians found this scent the least appealing.

CALLING ALL WANNABE LESBIANS: THE STRAIGHT GIRL'S GUIDE TO SEX WITH A WOMAN

Bi-curiosity – women sleeping with women simply because they want to know what it's like – is increasingly common, and rather than being frowned upon it's seen as seriously cool. Madonna, Kate Moss, Pink and Naomi Campbell are all rumoured to have had lesbian flingettes. And every sane woman in the entire world puts her hand up and says, 'Yes please,' when asked if they'd like to take a girly tumble with the straight girl's fantasy queen, Angelina Jolie. Sex guru Kinsey claimed that by the age of thirty, one woman in four has felt sexually attracted to another woman. By age forty, he claims, one in five have consummated a lesbian relationship. Recent reliable statistics are hard to come by (even if the participants aren't finding it hard to come) because a fair amount of women feel embarrassed owning up to their fantasies or experiences. Through my writing and research, and through talking with lesbian friends, I consider Kinsey's estimates to be way too low. I know lots of straight women who not only have pretty hot fantasies, they claim they'd act on them if the situation arose. I figure that if they're thinking about it, the chances are lots of you are too, and perhaps it would be a good idea to address a few of the issues you may have. So here you go: this is a first timer's guide to sleeping with a woman, compiled and approved by a selection of bi-curious, bisexual and lesbian women.

STICKY FINGERS: TOUCHING TECHNIQUES WHICH WORK ON EVERY WOMAN

- **Double up:** Cross your middle finger over your index finger and slide your fingers in and out of her vagina, twisting like a screw. With the other hand, make quick circles around her clitoris, adding lube if she feels dry.
- **Put the pressure on:** Put lots of lube on the pads of your fingers and make circles around her clitoris. Start off with big, slow circles, making them smaller and faster as you continue. Vary the pressure of your fingertips: start lightly with the big circles and increase the pressure for the smaller ones. Change direction occasionally.
- **Walk the walk:** Pretend your fingers are two legs and gently 'walk' up and down her clitoral area, wiggling your fingers as you go.
- **Get behind her:** Get her to sit with her legs spread wide open, then sit behind her, with your legs on the outside of hers. From behind, use one hand to stimulate her breasts and the other to work on her clitoris. You can also kiss at the same time.

- **What's different about sleeping with a woman, compared to a man?** The first thing you'll probably notice is how soft and smooth women feel. Doing it to someone who has what you have feels strange but it's also comforting: you feel you've got a bit of a head start compared to the first time you slept with a man. When you're touching or licking her, knowing what it would feel like if it was being done to you is an erotic extra. Like gay men, you'll notice that women switch sexual roles much more than straight couples do. You'll tend not to split into 'giver' and 'taker', you both take turns. Because women take longer to orgasm than men do, you may find women are more patient and you feel less pressure to hurry up and orgasm. One woman said it felt incredibly safe. Oh, and you can both have *lots* of orgasms rather than just one, so there's no definite ending to a sex session.

> 'Not once did I orgasm with a man but I still had no idea I was gay – I'd never met any gay girls before. The first time I did, my eyes met this girl's and I felt a jolt and thought, that's odd. Two weeks later I woke up in the middle of the night and realized, my God, I'm gay. It explained my whole life to me.'
>
> Lauren, 30

- **Where do I go to meet gay women?** If you've got gay girlfriends, simply tag along with them to a lesbian bar. If you don't, it can be a bit intimidating walking in on your own ('It felt a bit like I had a neon sign above my head saying virgin. It was incredibly cliquey to begin with,' said one girl.) Some women said you should think about what you'll wear since this will reflect how you want to be treated. If you dress feminine and pretty, you'll be the 'girl'; turn up in masculine clothes and you'll be the 'boy'. Others said this was a load of old bollocks and you shouldn't pigeonhole yourself.

As for who to approach, the kind of lesbian you pick is probably going to determine what kind of experience you have. 'If you go for someone very feminine, you're probably going to have a soft, girly experience – kind of like sleeping with one of your girlfriends, only more experienced,' said one girl who recommends sleeping with someone butch the first time. 'They look scary but they usually aren't and if you don't know what to do, they're likely to take charge. Often, they don't expect or even want anything in return. If you're a bit squeamish when it comes to going down on a girl, this can be a good thing.'

If you don't like the idea of going to a bar, flick through a lesbian magazine – they're available in most countries or you can find them by searching the net – and see what gay events there are. Even easier, go on line and cruise the many lesbian websites on offer in each country. Lots are used by straight women who want to hook up with a lesbian. Another alternative is to look in a gay-friendly newspaper and answer a personal ad. Or you could just hang around your gay friends for a bit and see who you get introduced to. Go with what feels comfortable.

> 'It's incredibly rare to not have an orgasm girl-on-girl. But it's incredibly common for straight girls not to have one with their man.'
>
> Stacey, 28

- **Do lesbians even like sleeping with straight women?** This is an interesting one. While lots of gay men say they fantasize about sex with a straight guy, women aren't so keen, to the point where three of the girls I interviewed had to lie to get laid for the first time. 'All the gay girls I know have no interest in straight women and the ones who do inevitably end up with their hearts broken,' said one girl. Another friend said she 'wouldn't go there with a barge pole. They'd have to be superhot for me to take the risk. She's likely to either go back to her boyfriend or discover she's gay and want to experiment with other women – either way you can't win!'

'You don't ever want to be anyone's first,' was something I heard over and over. Others were more worried about breaking *her* heart. 'Women are so clingy and needy and once you've blown their minds – and you do because, let's face it, lesbian sex is the best sex out there – she's going to be all emotional and you're never going to get rid of her.' Which leaves you in a bit of a spot: if you take the advice of the people I've spoken to, you won't admit you're straight or that it's your first time. You may have to lie, in other words, which some of you may not be prepared to do. The alternative is to simply say nothing and if they bring up the topic say, 'I'm kind of shy talking about sex.'

> **❶ Do gay dads end up with gay sons? In a word, no. The largest ever study of gay fathers and straight sons found that only 9 per cent turned out to be gay – further evidence that homosexuality is not environmentally transmitted.**

- **What if I'm just having sex to satisfy my curiosity?** Should you tell her? Again, it's a damned-if-you-do, damned-if-you-don't thing. Most of the girls I spoke to said of course you should tell, but that might mean they won't go there. Straight women I spoke to all said they would confess. The same women, incidentally, who usually have no qualms about using a guy for sex. So why think twice when it's sex with a woman? It's because we perceive women to attach more feelings to sex than men do. This is quite right in a lot of cases, but anyone who's ever tuned into *The L Word* and watched Shane attach her lips and hips to around ten women a week, knows there are women out there who will be very happy to shag and leave you. 'I sometimes just fancy someone and want to have sex with that person whether she's gay or straight,' said one girl. 'If she's quite an alpha female with men, she'll probably be good in bed with a girl.'

> 'One of my really close friends told me she'd slept with a woman while on holiday. She'd always fancied doing it but was scared people would find out. By doing it with a stranger in another country, she got to indulge without the post-sex paranoia.'
>
> Anna, 31

- **How do I suggest going to bed?** Flirt a bit, touch a little longer and more sexually than you would usually, stand close, make lots of eye contact and . . . hang on, doesn't this sound familiar? Dead right, it's the same way you'd show a man you're interested. Except, unlike with a man, if she knows you're straight you're probably going to have to make all the moves. 'I'd flirt a little to test the water, but I'd let her make the definitive move. I wouldn't want to push her, misread the situation or be blamed for taking advantage of a weak moment,' said one girl.

If you fancy someone in a bar, it's late, they've had more than two sips of sherry and there seems to be lots of snogging going on, they may assume you're gay and move in on you too. So if you're going to be shocked by a forward approach (i.e. a tongue in your mouth and hand up your jumper) best speak up fairly quickly. Say something like, 'Hi, I'm new to all this, seems like fun though,' quite early on. If you've answered an ad, there's no need to say anything at all. You've already done that simply by replying.

- **Will she be able to tell if I've never slept with a woman before?** Five of the girls I interviewed said they'd pretended to be experienced with their first female lover and got away with it. 'It can be done. If you like sex generally and are into it, it probably won't be a problem.' So long as you're adventurous and assertive, most women probably wouldn't be able to tell you're a virgin, but they might well figure it out

According to Kinsey, between 62 and 79 per cent of men who say they're gay have had sex with women.

afterwards. 'I'd spot it immediately by her emotional reaction,' said one. 'First-timers are often overemotional after the sex is over.'

THE KINSEY SCALE

The 'Kinsey Scale' was invented by the infamous sexologist to measure how gay someone is. 'Totally straight' people scored 0, 'totally gay' got you a six. Everyone else fell somewhere in between the two, depending on what they got up to and wanted to get up to. Rather than branding people, Kinsey invented the scale to demonstrate how fluid our sexuality is. It's rumoured the man himself rated 1 when he first opened the Kinsey Institute but soared to 5 or 6 later in life.

- **Worried about how you'll perform?** Don't commit the classic first-timers mistake of assuming you'll know exactly what she likes just because she's got what you've got. We're all individual, and what makes your eyes roll back in ecstasy could make her roll her eyes to the ceiling in boredom or frustration. On the other hand, if you're stuck for inspiration, think about what turns you on. After all, all that's happening is you're on a different side to all the techniques guys used on you. If you're really nervous, simply say, 'I don't know what to do. Will you take charge?' And lie back and enjoy . . . though not for long: 'lazy girls' aren't a huge hit with lesbians! Practice makes perfect, but it wouldn't hurt to read up a little on the topic of lesbian sex. Choose from one of the many excellent books available, but don't get *too* caught up in needing to be good in bed. As the saying goes, 'Sex is perfectly natural, it's not naturally perfect'.

SAME SEX SAFE SEX

OK, here's the deal. Anyone who has read any of my other books knows I am a strong advocate of safe sex. I'm also well aware that the official guidelines are rigid and people often choose to ignore some of the recommendations and make what they consider to be sensible decisions.

I'm going to list everything you should be doing, then it's up to you to decide what risks you want to take. Quite honestly, the only real guaranteed defence against all STIs is not to have sex at all – condoms can't protect you against everything – but the second best defence is to use common sense, know the facts about safe sex, what's dangerous and what's not, then make sensible decisions based on your particular relationship. Don't drink excessively or do drugs and you've got a chance of actually remembering what decisions you made. Here are the basics you should know:

- For men, condoms used properly and every single time are still your best protection at this point. They will protect you against STIs spread by the exchange of bodily fluids – sperm, blood, mucus etc. – but you can still catch herpes and warts because they can be spread simply by touching infected skin. Pubic lice and scabies will jump merrily onto pubic hair no matter how many condoms you have on.

- Kissing is relatively low-risk for most things, including HIV transmission, but you can contract herpes if the person has a cold sore on their mouth.
- Oral sex is less risky than anal sex, as long as neither of you have cuts, abrasions or scratches. The trouble is they're often tiny and unnoticeable. To be truly safe you should ensure that the person you're giving oral sex to wears a condom. If you choose not to, be aware that allowing someone to ejaculate in your mouth increases the risk of transmission of some STIs and swallowing the semen ups it further. Lesbians should also be aware that although the risk is low, it's still a good idea to put a piece of cling film or cut-up condom between your mouth and their genitals.
- Rimming (licking someone's anus) puts you at risk of Hepatitis A and B, among other things. You'd be advised to use cling film or a cut-up condom to cover the anus during rimming and wear latex gloves for fisting.
- Anal sex minus a condom continues to be the highest-risk sexual activity for HIV transmission. You seriously need to be armed with more than a glint in your eye, i.e. strong condoms and a good lubricant so they're less likely to tear.

Generally, there's a lot more foreplay before you actually get to the bedroom because women are more tactile and touchy-feely than men. Once you're into it, there's a heavy concentration on kissing, lots of breast play and fingering and (you guessed it) tons of oral sex. Scissoring – rubbing your crotch area up against each other – sometimes features, vibrators generally don't (women are better at giving other women orgasms, so there's no need).

Depending on whether you're with a 'vanilla' lesbian (not wildly adventurous) or a person who's into hard-core sex, fisting is unlikely to feature first time round, though a strap-on dildo might.

- **Does it mean I'm gay if I want a repeat performance?** Almost all the women I spoke with said you know if you're really gay the second you sleep with a woman. It's an entirely different feeling than simply enjoying it. Some women insist occasional lesbians are in denial, but lots agree that there are women who are mainly straight but enjoy the odd dabble. You will probably think about it a lot though, either way. Just as your first time with a man affects you deeply, so does your first time with a woman and your connection with this girl will be strong. You may feel guilty if you've cheated on a boyfriend or weird if you liked it. If you liked it more than you like sex with men and felt a sense of relief or as if you'd 'come home' you might want to get those pretty little hands of yours on some books that talk about lesbian coming-out stories and see if you identify with them. There's lots of support if you do decide you're gay – Google 'lesbian support groups' and you'll find plenty.

HOW TO USE A STRAP-ON

Straight women use them to anally penetrate their boyfriends, lesbians use them to penetrate each other. If you've never used a strap-on dildo, you probably think they look scary or even faintly ridiculous – OK, seriously ridiculous. I have to confess, I wore one to indulge an ex-boyfriend once, but got so carried away with strutting around imagining what it would be like to be a well-hung stud that we sort of missed the moment. Regular users who actually get around to inserting them swear they're the best invention for penetrative sex since God invented the penis. You'd like to try using one but aren't sure how? Keep reading. Everything you need to know is right here.

For her to use on her: There's an urban myth that if you want penetration, you're not really a lesbian because you obviously miss a penis. This makes about as much sense as saying anyone who likes listening to 'Big Spender' secretly wants to be a stripper. Most women enjoy being penetrated during sex for one simple reason: it feels good. Fingers, penis, vibrator, dildo or the carrot you'd been saving for that stew – it doesn't really matter what, except that there are obvious advantages to using a dildo: for a start it never goes soft. The experience of 'fucking someone' – as most of my lesbian friends delicately put it – is incredibly erotic. It's a power rush and you feel naughty and edgy doing it. Best of all, you get to pick exactly what length and thickness suits you, while straight women obviously don't. (You could try choosing your men by getting them all to drop their trousers but I think you'll find the man attached to the penis will insist on being involved as well.)

Dildos are the world's oldest sex toys, so not surprisingly there are loads to choose from. Once you've chosen one, or several, dildos to suit you, pick a harness to suit. You can hold the dildo in your hand but a harness means your hands are free to stimulate other bits. The standard model has straps that go around your thighs and another around your waist. The dildo is either already attached or fits into a pocket. It's a very good idea to practise wearing a strap-on *before* trying it out with your partner, just in case you, like me, get a fit of the giggles or feel silly. Some women roll a condom on the dildo for hygiene reasons and most use lube as well. ➢

Unlike normal intercourse, it's the person on the receiving end who is in charge during strap-on sex. The reason why is that a penis has nerve endings, a dildo doesn't, so the wearer has no idea how deep they're going. Make it pleasurable rather than painful by speaking up and being specific about what you'd like – a slow, circular grind or hard thrust etc. The person wearing the harness usually orgasms by positioning the straps or base of the dildo so it's rubbing on their clitoris. Some harnesses include a small pouch designed to hold a small vibrator in just the right spot or you could slip on a vibrating penis ring (see page 283), turning it round to work on you, rather than your partner. As with penis penetration, she'll need foreplay first and is likely to get just as bored as straight women do if you go on and on and on.

For her to use on him: Being penetrated by a woman is a novel experience for a guy, since he's normally the one poking things into holes. It's not something regularly requested by a lot of men, so I really wouldn't surprise him on his birthday by disappearing to the bathroom and emerging with a huge lifelike dildo strapped over that delicate, wispy thong. It's one thing having a tongue, finger or even a teensy weensy vibrator inserted anally, it's quite another having a full-size penis. For a start, he's got to be sexually secure enough not to panic that it will make him gay. Secondly, you need to build up to anal sex with a dildo in the same way you would for anal sex with a penis.

Follow the same rules listed in the anal sex guide on pages 104–6, then hold the base of the dildo before inserting it slowly and shallowly at first. Just one other word of warning: not all men want to try this doggie style, as in you behind them. Some guys like lying on their back, with their legs in the air, adopting the female role in the good old missionary position. This totally freaks out some women because it's a little too girly. If you notice she's started to lock her underwear drawer, stick to doing it from behind.

FISTING FOR FIRST-TIMERS

I'm sorry, but as much as I'm going to faithfully and diligently report all the ins and outs on this one, I'm *so* not going to be speaking from experience. There's something about fisting – well, everything about fisting – which makes me want to cross my legs *very* tightly and put both hands over my bits and keep them there – for ever! My lesbian and some of my straight, friends assure me that done properly it doesn't hurt, but until you hear otherwise (like see an announcement on my website saying, 'Tried fisting last night and do you know what, guys? You're right, it's fabulous!') assume I am still a fisting virgin. Rest assured, though, my fisting friends – did I really just say that? – have checked my research and assured me it's all accurate. So here goes. All of this information, by the way, is for both straights and lesbians. Fisting isn't particularly mainstream behaviour for any sexual group, but it appears to be *marginally* more common among lesbians than others, hence it appearing here.

> 'Fisting for us isn't premeditated. It's something which happens when you're so turned on and wet that you go with the flow. My girlfriend and I have never even had to use lubricant.'
>
> Heather, 33

CAN YOU TELL BY SOMEONE'S HANDS WHETHER THEY ARE GAY OR STRAIGHT?

Now here's an answer you probably weren't expecting: it's possible. Recent research suggests that lesbians have ➤

a 91 per cent greater chance of being left-handed or ambidextrous than straight women and also have a ring finger which is longer than their index finger – the opposite to the average straight woman's finger ratio. Gay men are 34 per cent more likely to be lefties than straights. The connection between left-handedness and homosexuality was discovered by researchers who analysed twenty different studies done over the past fifty years.

More and more research seems to suggest our sexual orientation is in the genes, and we appear to be most affected during the period in the womb when our fingers form. If people are exposed to a high level of testosterone during this time, scientists think it may wire the brain for attraction to the same sex. It also affects finger length, which is why lots of researchers believe relative finger length is a marker for sexuality which has been moulded by hormones. Straight men tend to have ring fingers slightly longer than their index finger. For straight women, they're the same length or the index is just a bit longer.

A longer ring finger than your index finger appears to say 'testosterone was here'. Females with masculine finger ratios tend to display more blokey behaviour than women who don't, while men with the female ratio – index longer than ring finger – are more in touch with their female side. The correct way to measure your fingers, by the way, is to measure from the crease of each finger to the tip, palm side. Interesting as it is, this research is by no means definitive, so play nicely, boys and girls. No accusing your partner of being secretly straight/gay if the finger ratio doesn't match their sexual orientation.

- **Do you really trust the person you're about to do it with?** Let's face it, though we all know babies come out of one end and sometimes astonishingly enormous poos out of the other, anyone who hasn't had a fist up either orifice would understandably have to *really* trust their partner to want to give it a shot.
- **There is a right way to do it:** Just like anal sex, you need to follow a procedure rather than dive straight in.

Rule No 1: Don't do it for the first time while drunk or on drugs as you need to be completely aware of what you're doing. Both also tend to numb the area, so what feels bloody marvellous at the time hurts like hell the next day.

> 'It was awful. I went to put my finger inside and my whole hand disappeared. Everything felt *way* too extended.'
>
> Jo, 18

Rule No 2: It may feel uncomfortable, especially the first few times, but it shouldn't *really* hurt. Stop if it does and if there is any sign of blood. Some of my friends say a little bit of blood is quite normal, but I'm sticking with the no-blood-allowed theory.

Rule No 3: Again like anal sex, this isn't something you're going to accomplish in one sex session. Have patience and remember, practice makes perfect, and sometimes it's just not possible. Some women's vaginas are just too small and the hands too big and some people's bottoms just can't cope with it.

The step-by-step guide to vaginal fisting

Em and Lo from www.nerve.com provide a brilliant step-by-step guide in *The Big Bang*. I've taken some of their tips and combined them with other tried-and-tested techniques approved by friends and other sources to come up with this basic guide:

- **Check your hands and nails don't have any rough spots:** Take off any rings, bracelets, watches etc.
- **Pull on a pair of unpowdered latex gloves:** They make it easier to enter and exit and also help stop the spread of disease. Add *lots* of lube, and continue to add it throughout if needed.
- **Get into position and indulge in some foreplay:** She'll need to be aroused for her vagina to expand. Once you're done that, get her to lie on her back with her knees bent and prop yourself up on your elbows and knees.
- **Start with one finger:** Slowly work up to two, three, four fingers, then, if she says she's ready, press your fingers together like you're imitating a duck bill to make your hand as narrow and small as possible, then begin to insert your hand, palm facing up and thumb folded in.
- **Get your partner to breathe deeply:** She should breathe out and bear down with her vaginal muscles, as if she were if pushing out a baby, so she feels in control.
- **Rotate your hand slightly:** moving it back and forth until it enters the vagina then form a tight fist, keeping your thumb tucked in.
- **Hold still:** Ohmigod, you've done it. You're inside. You're probably feeling mighty turned on, she's feeling mighty vulnerable. Hold perfectly still until she says she's happy for you to move.
- **Make small movements:** The bigger the object you're inserting, the smaller and gentler the movement. Try slightly twisting your fist or gently clenching and unclenching it. Thrust back and forth only when she's feeling completely comfortable.

- **Add more lube:** If you think wet fisting sounds painful, imagine what it would feel like if she gets dry.
- **Prepare to exit when you've both had enough:** tell her you're about to exit, so she can prepare by bearing down and breathing deeply. Leave her slowly and gently by reversing all the instructions you followed to get in there in the first place. Even if she panics and suddenly wants you to *get outta there*, don't pull out suddenly. Agree instantly to stop but still remove your hand slowly and gracefully.

The step-by-step guide to anal fisting

Read the above, it all pretty much applies, except that you have to be even more careful. Vaginas are used to things popping in and out of them – penises, tampons, babies, vibrators – bottoms tend not to see as much incoming traffic. Other differences: vaginas lubricate, bottoms don't, vaginas are elastic, bottoms aren't as much. You need to double the lube and do double the checking all is OK for it all to go smoothly.

> 'Admitting you're gay is a process, not an event. Mostly because you don't want it to be true. So even after you've done something with another guy the denial/survival mechanism kicks in. I slept with a couple of guys and *totally* denied I was gay for a long time.'
>
> John, 40

- **Get in training:** Start inserting a finger inside the anus on a regular basis, then work up to using an anal vibrator or dildo. Only ever insert ones with a flared base or you might be in for one of those trips to the emergency ward we all scoff at when news gets out – and it will. The point when your partner is ready for fisting anally, according to experts, is when they can comfortably take a dildo which is around three inches wide.

- **Get into the doggie position and follow all the above steps for vaginal fisting:** Take into account all the above warnings. It's crucial you talk to your partner during penetration. Ask them if it's OK to push in further before you move a muscle or theirs could spasm painfully.
- **Expect it to take time to reach your goal:** As Em and Lo wisely say, 'Don't expect to get your whole hand in the first time. Don't expect to get your whole hand in the fifteenth time.' N.B.: A word of warning for any fisters, back or front door: It's suggested you wait a few days before having intercourse vaginally and anally in case you've torn the lining of both. See, it's things like this which make me want to go 'Ow' and 'Ewww', but best of luck to all you brave people out there who are planning on giving it a go.

> 'The best thing about being a gay man is understanding and liking the competitiveness of straight men but also having this immense love for and connection with women that goes way beyond what straight males feel.'
>
> John, 36

MAN TO MAN: THE STRAIGHT GUY'S GUIDE TO HAVING SEX WITH A MAN

Society watches lasciviously when women fool around with other women, but a man who decides to have a same-sex experience isn't treated with the same indulgence. Walk into a dodgy bar late at night and you're more than likely to find some tipsy girls French kissing in an attempt to entice men. Few straight men would pull that stunt, and even if they did, it wouldn't work because most women say they're either repulsed or unaffected by men having a snog. Instead of flaunting a tryst with the same sex, as plenty of women do, most straight guys hide it in the emotional equivalent of a three-feet-deep steel chest surrounded by starving Rottweilers, an alarm system and a moat. Because, as I said, despite a definite relaxation of the homophobic hype surrounding lesbians, this hasn't translated to gay men. Rumours about being secretly gay are still the stuff of nightmares, which is why a man who wants to have a one-off encounter with another man will think much longer and harder about it than a woman would. Either that or he won't think about it at all, do it on the spur of the moment and spend years agonizing over what happened.

What's different about sleeping with a man, compared to a woman? Well, there's no need to wine or dine, make small talk or (heaven!) pretend to be interested in the then-he-said, then-she-said stuff she comes out with. Gay men tend to be more honest and direct about sex, but don't buy into the myth that promiscuity is the norm. 'If you're in a sex club, bathhouse or the back room of a very seedy bar, cutting straight to the chase, like staring at someone's crotch or grabbing it, is acceptable,' says a friend of mine. 'But if you're in a classy club or bar, it's a turn-off and you'll be seen as a bit of a jerk.'

Gay men are more likely to be well hung than straight guys. The average length of a gay man's erect penis is 6.32 inches, while straights only clock up 5.99 inches. Researchers suspect it's the result of a 'hypermasculine' effect of androgen hormones in the womb, which they also think is responsible for making men gay.

'My defining moment, the moment I knew for sure, was when I found myself in a gay bar, picked up a guy, spent the night and it just felt so *right*. It wasn't just that the sex was great – it wasn't – it was the comfort of being with another man in an affectionate way.'

Scott, 23

Unless it's long term, there's less emotional investment for men, so there's less talking. Because men get aroused quicker than women do, sex is quicker. It's primal and you're able to let go and suggest all those kinky fantasies without fear of offending.

Where do I go to meet gay men? All the men I spoke to said a gay club is your best bet. But again, don't buy into the myth that just because you're a man, a gay man will automatically want to have his wicked way with you. As one person put it: 'Gay men are portrayed as being willing to have sex anytime, any place and with anyone. The first two I tend to agree with, but the 'anyone' couldn't be further from the truth. Do you have any idea how picky gay men are about appearance? If there's one myth that couldn't be further from the truth, it's the one that says just because you're male, we'll sleep with you.'

It's also wishful thinking that picking up a man, or getting picked up by one, is simply a case of walking across a bar and saying, 'Hi, you're hot. How about it?' Most will hit on you in much the same way you'd hit on her: 'Can I buy you a drink?'; lots of eye contact; 'accidental', lingering touches – all the moves you used on her will probably be used on you.

If you want to do the initiating, start up a general conversation, send out some signals as above, then if you think they're interested say, 'This bar/club is way too loud, do you want to go somewhere quieter?' Quieter could mean another bar, coffee, your place or his. Once you are somewhere private and it's obvious you're both massively attracted, this is where it does differ from being with a female. Rather than

> 'People assume all gay men have anal sex, but in reality lots of us don't. I've never been penetrated and have no intention of letting it happen. Hands, mouths and tongues do the job more than adequately.'
>
> Richard, 42

pretending to be interested in her cat and stretching out the sex thing into several (long) nights – first night a snog, second night breasts, third night third base etc. – it's perfectly acceptable and expected to have sex within an hour or so of arriving there. If you want to take it slow, confess. Say, 'Look, I've only ever slept with women but feel attracted to men, so I'm not really sure what's going to happen tonight'. Some men won't be interested if you're not a sure thing, others may tread carefully emotionally if they're looking for a long-term relationship, but if you're good looking, I strongly suspect you won't be short of offers.

'What's the worst thing about being a gay man? The lack of tolerance and destroying your parents' idealistic vision of how your life could be.'

Rob, 23

Do gay men like seducing straight men? Like gay women who circle straights suspiciously, most of the gay men I spoke to were also wary. 'It's the fear of physical harm – approach the wrong guy and you could be in real trouble,' one man said. Other reasons why you might not be top of their wish list are that other gay men accept them for who they are, you may not; you're just out for a shag and they may be looking for a relationship; they'll probably have to work hard to seduce you and it's often not worth it. Some guys say that at the end of the day, a lot of straight guys lie there expecting to be serviced.

> ❶ *Research backs up what everyone secretly thinks: self-confessed homophobes are far more likely to be aroused by footage showing gay men having sex than straight guys.*

Having said that, I've watched lots of my gay male friends flirt with my straight ones, and vice versa. On the other hand, I flirt with gay men, gay women, straight men, straight

Around one-third of all US males are thought to have had at least one same-sex experience leading to orgasm since puberty compared to around half of college-educated women.

women, dogs, cats and budgies but that doesn't mean I want to have sex with them. So opinion divides on whether seducing a virgin is a good experience or not. 'You definitely get a buzz from knowing you're the first, and it's a huge turn-on watching how turned on he is, but he'll often come way too fast and the minute the sex is over lots of straight men have a strong emotional gut reaction about what they've just done,' said one friend, echoing the words of many.

Prominent US gay columnist, TV presenter and very good friend Michael Alvear agrees about the emotional fallout. 'My first time involved lots of fumbling, not really knowing what to do and being grossed out and turned on at the same time. Grossed out because I didn't want to be gay and turned on because I was. I'd say it was the worst and best sex ever. Worst in terms of technique but best in terms of the high.' Put simply, you're liable to act weird afterwards and that's not always pleasant to be around.

'When I told my sister, I cried like a baby. There is something about verbalizing it – saying "I'm gay" – that cements it. I took so long to get it out, she burst out crying saying, "Thank God! I thought you were going to tell me you had inoperable cancer."'

Tim, 31

What if I'm just having sex to satisfy my curiosity? Should I tell him? If you're picking up a guy in a club for a night of hot sex, there's no real need to. In fact, they'd probably think you were bonkers if you *did* start apologizing that sex is all you want. If you've met the guy through different circumstances and think he might be up for a relationship rather than a one-nighter, steer clear or make your intentions known. 'Whether you confess totally depends on the venue,' says one friend. 'I assume men in bars or clubs are out to get laid, but if I met a guy through some friends at a party at his place, I'd be far more likely to think about considering them for a relationship.'

Can he tell if I've never slept with a man before? Most probably, though he may think it's just nerves, lack of experience or, worse, bad technique that's affecting your performance. But if you're having sex to find out if you're gay, rather than giving in to an experimental urge, it's likely the experience will be so emotional he's unlikely to miss it. Another friend said that 'My first time was absolutely horrible. My heart was bumping so hard that I thought it would jump out of my chest. My whole body was shaking and I felt very uncomfortable. I think I wanted it too much and that's why my body reacted the opposite way – it was the guilt feeling that took all the pleasure away.'

What does a typical gay-men sex session involve? Gay men are more active than straight couples, they'll roll around and change sides and positions a lot more than a man and woman. They're also not shy about telling you what they want. Some men like kissing, others don't. You'll probably start by masturbating yourself and each other, and you may be surprised to see he uses a completely different technique to you. Men are very specific about masturbation, and technique depends on the size of his penis and personal preference. The trick to getting it right when you do it to him is to position your fingers where he does at the *start*, then simply imitate what he did. Men don't have in-built lubricants like your girlfriend did, so you'll need to add lubrication. (A little pre-ejaculatory fluid is produced but not massive amounts.) Your girlfriend may have looked disgusted, but it's totally acceptable to spit on your hand or drip some on his penis.

After mutual manual masturbation, you'll probably move into giving and receiving oral sex. Unlike women, who can't see what's really happening when it's done to them, you have had a bird's-eye view of what previous female lovers got up to down there, so there's no need to be nervous. Put one hand around the base of his penis to hold it steady, then do what she did if that sensation felt good. Don't attempt to take him too deeply into your mouth the first time. If you feel like gagging, move his penis to the side of your mouth or concentrate on the head. Few gay men swallow, and not just because it's unsafe. They, like you, like watching penises ejaculate. Some gay men then move on to some form of anal stimulation, either rimming (see page 233), inserting a finger or full anal sex (see pages 104–6 for a guide on how to have safe anal sex). Don't be alarmed if you suddenly feel a quick slap on your bottom during it, by the way. Gay men call them 'love taps' and a sexy spank is quite common in gay sex.

Does it mean I'm gay if I want a repeat performance? The gay men I spoke to answered this question the same way the lesbians did: you'll know if you're gay the minute you sleep with a man. You might decide to deny or ignore it, but it will be clear. Some men decide to remain straight but have occasional sex with other men – usually strangers they've picked up randomly. I don't need to point out the moral dilemmas you may wrangle with if you choose this option. If you decide instead that you're predominantly gay, do what I've suggested for women. Google 'gay support groups' and you'll see there's lots of advice to help you make the transition from straight to gay, if you want to.

Be careful! I've never heard of a lesbian being physically hurt simply because she liked women, but a good friend of mine almost got killed by a gang of thugs a couple of years ago for walking into a gay bar. 'The danger is so pronounced that most gay guys live in a low-level state of anticipatory anxiety,'

HANDLING HIM: TRICKS ANY PENIS WILL ADORE

- **Get comfy:** The best way to manipulate him isn't side-by-side. Instead, lie on your back with your knees bent and get him to straddle your stomach on his knees. Both of you get a great view and he can work on you at the same time.

- **Switch sensations:** No matter how good a technique feels, our bodies rapidly become desensitized – you really can have too much of a good thing. Try alternating a fast, firm touch with a slower, softer one, switching between the two every few minutes. Do this at the start to maximize feeling, concentrating more on the fast, firmer stroke as he gets closer to orgasm.

- **Switch sides:** Instead of focusing on the whole shaft, stimulate one side of his penis at a time. Start with one hand holding the penis around the base, fingers flat on his pubic hair. Wrap your other hand around the base of his penis, then let it glide smoothly up to the head letting your palm massage the head, before sliding down the opposite side. Don't let your hand lose contact at any point and don't be frightened to take a good, firm grip.

- **Finish the job properly:** According to gay men, women are rubbish when it comes to hand-job finales. We either stop too soon or go too heavy too long. The correct way to take him through to a seamless climax is to stroke quickly as he approaches orgasm, using firm pressure and without loosening your hold. As you feel the start of his orgasm – his testicles lift toward his body and you can feel contractions as the semen is ejaculated – lighten your strokes. Stop completely when the semen stops coming out.

he says. 'We're constantly thinking how gay-friendly our environment is. My boyfriend and I hold hands, but we'll drop them simultaneously when we sense it's going to put us at risk, either socially or physically. The fact that we do it at same time without words passing between us shows how deep the fear is and how fine-tuned our radars are.'

While a female tends to dabble in same-sex scenarios with few or pleasurable consequences, a man experimenting with a man can suffer strong emotional and physical repercussions.

DO SAME-SEX MARRIAGES DIFFER FROM STRAIGHT MARRIAGES?

While there are loads of studies on gay and lesbian sex and umpteen theories as to why some people are straight and others gay, scientists aren't quite so keen to study their long-term relationships – whoever said white-coat researchers are nerds was wrong: they're all sex mad! We know from an old study that gay men, who've been able to marry since 1989 in Denmark, stay together much longer than straight Danish couples – 17 per cent of divorces for gay men compared to 46 per cent for straight couples. The stats for female hook-ups is less impressive, though still applaudable by comparison – only 23 per cent of lesbian marriages fail – exactly half that of straight couples.

One study in 2004 suggests that longevity isn't the only lesson straights can learn from gay marriages; housework and childcare is far more equitable in same-sex unions as well. This survey compared gay men and lesbians in civil unions in the US with married straights and found domestic chores to be far more equally shared among the gay couples. Straight couples tend to share the chores early on but slip into traditional roles – she does all the housework as he sits with his feet up watching telly – once they marry. (Any female teetering on the edge of coming out: this may well convince you!)

8 Ask Me Anything

The most asked, most embarrassing, most peculiar sex questions

●●

Being known as a 'sexpert' has its perks (can you think of something more interesting to specialize in?) but it also has its drawbacks. Like when you're out at a pub or restaurant, half-sloshed, headed for the loo and concentrating fiercely on balancing on your heels, only to be waylaid by someone who's decided now's the perfect time to finally find out the answer to something that's puzzled them for years. Most of the time I'm more than happy to pontificate, but sometimes (like when my eyeballs are spinning around with the effort of having to focus) it's a lot simpler to promise to send someone a book. If it's you I meet on the way to the loo, you can bet it's this book and this chapter I'll be directing you to. This is a selection of the type of stuff I'm usually asked, and a few quirky questions I couldn't resist including because they really did make me smile.

My ex used to love me to pull her hair during sex and get a little rough. I loved doing it but am too scared to suggest it to my new girlfriend for fear she'll think I'm odd.

If your girlfriend is a feisty, lusty female rather than a prudish, squeamish girly-girl, it's unlikely to shock her. She might not be into it, but it's not dodgy enough to make her look at you with new, horrified eyes. Loads of females are into hair-pulling and mock force. It feeds into the primitive part of our brain that wants Me-Jane, You-Tarzan sex and it overrides the nice-girls-don't thing – though it does not, I repeat, does *not*, indicate any desire for a man to be violent.

Sex and pain have always been linked, which is why we often leave love bites and back scratches behind. How to suggest it? The next time you're having sex and kissing, grab her hair to make a ponytail in one hand and hold it quite tightly. If there's no adverse reaction, tug it gently so she's forced to lift her chin and expose her throat, which naturally you'll ravish with your lips and tongue.

Does she lean into you and seem aroused? Or say, 'Ouch!' and glare at you. If women don't like 'rough', most will let you know about it.

If the hair-pulling goes well, try putting your hands around her waist and pulling her quite forcefully towards you down the bed. Another green light, she's up for it, but it's wise to keep on checking she's happy during any type of 'rough' sex, especially at the start.

I read somewhere that men like vibrators used on them. But how and where and how do I suggest it?
If you're going to use it on him, let him use it on you first. Wait until you're both in a wicked mood and having hot and heavy foreplay, then say, 'Hey, do you want to use my vibrator?' and deftly reach into your bedside drawer and fish it out. What he claps his eyes on, by the way, shouldn't be a 'rabbit' or anything styled to look like a real penis. A small wand vibrator – the simple sort, long and cylindrical – is the least threatening for a first time. Don't be surprised if you get

a lukewarm response – lots of men are secretly terrified they'll be replaced by something far more efficient at inducing female orgasm – and they'd be right, it is. This is why it's important you get him to use it on you first time, rather than expertly showing him how you can orgasm in around a minute (it'll crush all his sexual pride in about the same time, since it takes him fifteen minutes on a good day).

Once he's played around, it's fairly easy to cheerfully say, 'Your turn,' grab it from him and quickly hone in on . . . his shoulders. Use it to soothe tense muscles and knots and the vibrator will be seen as his friend rather than public enemy No. 1. A little playful buzzing on the buttocks later and he'll soon be happy for you to try it on the perineum, the area between his anus and testicles. Put it on a low speed and press it firmly against the full length of this area, while you use your hand or mouth to simultaneously stimulate his penis. You could also try it at low speed on his anus: rub it in small circles around the outside but don't penetrate without lubrication and always wash it before putting it anywhere near your vagina afterwards. Another place to try is his testicles. Hold it underneath them and see what reaction you get. Some men *adore* this, but others would prefer you ripped each fingernail off one by one. Some men also like it rolled up and down the shaft of their penis, but in my experience this is the least favourite spot.

Is there any relationship between the size of a man's penis and how quickly he ejaculates?

Not only do below average-sized men have to grin and bear all those big-is-better jokes, they ejaculate much faster than their larger friends, so have to grit their teeth through jokes about that as well. Ha bloody ha, all right. All penises have roughly the same number of nerve endings in the head. If his penis is small, they're concentrated over a smaller area, which makes him more sensitive and prone to premature ejaculation. The opposite is true for men with big penises because the nerves are spread over a larger area. Highly unfair, yes, but there are lots of ways to deal with it. Become brilliant at oral sex, for instance, and the size of your penis becomes irrelevant. If you're really, *really* good she may not care if you have one at all.

How long does it take a woman to orgasm?

If you trip over your tongue just by looking at her, you've been snogging for England and it's the first time your hands have gone south, she might well orgasm in two minutes flat. If it's your partner of ten years, it might take two hours. Statistics vary wildly because it's something that's totally dependant on circumstances. Some say it takes twenty minutes for a woman to orgasm, others say eight minutes of direct clitoral stimulation will do the job. I think if the person knows which buttons to press and what works for you, eight to ten minutes sounds about right for oral or hand stimulation. That's on a good day, when everything else is favourable – hormones happy, not too much to drink, relationship going well, not stressing out about anything, having a 'thin' day, just bought a fab pair of shoes, the picture of her mother isn't in her line of vision . . .

> ❶ *53 per cent of Australian women admit to having a 'friend with benefits', a 'sex buddy' for regular but non-committed sex, at some stage in their lives. Far from being frowned upon, lots of experts applaud it, saying it's a much safer option than a typical one-night stand.*

My boyfriend calls his penis Arthur. What is all that about? Women don't name their bits, how come men do?

Frank, George, Wilbur, Arthur – men are fond of naming

their 'best friend', oddly, often by the very same names they use for their other best friend, the one with four legs. It all loops back to the male tendency to base their self-esteem on their masculinity and sexual prowess. Women usually base their self-worth on their relationships, men on qualities like strength, status, power and performance. The ultimate symbol of all of these, the penis, can therefore be quite terrifying to the man attached. Naming it makes it seem more friendly, softening the effect the penis has of, quite literally, holding its owner by the balls.

I like getting quite wild and noisy in bed but it seems to freak men out. Should I calm it down?

For every lover who shouts, 'Thank you *God*!' at the top of their lungs at the crucial moment, there's one who remains completely and utterly silent. If you're a loud, lusty girl in bed with an equally passionate vocal guy, feel free to wake up the people in the next county, though remember you may have to stand in line with them at the supermarket the next day. Shyer types may find your theatrics alarming – we distrust what we're not used to and shy tends to date shy and rowdy, rowdy. Others simply don't believe all that sheet-gripping and dramatic thrashing about is genuine and suspect you've seen one too many B-grade sex scenes. I'd play it safe at the start, then up the volume gradually.

I'm in love with a married man. Will he leave his wife for me?

Probably not, and even if he does it's unlikely it'll work out long term. Once the affair is out in the open, lots of people discover the appeal was the affair itself rather than the person. There's also a high level of mistrust because both of you know what each other is capable of. But that's assuming, rather optimistically, that he will leave. The chances are he won't because he's in a genuinely enviable position: his wife offers security and stability, you offer excitement and great sex, so why choose one when you can have both? He might tell you he's torn emotionally but the stark reality is that 44 per cent of men who have extramarital sex report slight or no emotional involvement. Only 11 per cent of women say the same.

The bottom line, however, is this: people have affairs to get something they're not getting from the relationship they're in. What's missing from his relationship with his wife is the crucial clue to finding your answer. Find out the real story: what do you give him that she doesn't? If it's something truly important and not just great fellatio, you might have a chance. One of the things people like best about affairs is that they get the chance to start over and be who they want to be, reinventing themselves. The more you make him feel he can be this person, 24/7, the more likely he is to want to leave. Then all you have to do is live with the guilt of having been instrumental in breaking up a marriage.

I recently dumped my boyfriend because I found out he'd slept with a prostitute. He was single at the time but it's completely put me off him. I don't understand why he would do that.

Politicians, actors, famous footballers, judges, doctors, City boys and half the men you and I know will probably visit a sex worker during their life. It's not desperation that sends them there but curiosity, among other things. Prostitutes are forbidden, i.e. a turn-on, he can do naughty things he wouldn't have dreamt of suggesting to you and it was no-strings sex. Instead of dumping him, perhaps you should have applauded his behaviour. It's a lot more honest than picking up some girl in a bar, having sex and never calling her again.

She's cheated on me once, but I've given her another chance. Am I right to trust her again?

Most definitely *not* if she's got a history of being unfaithful and being forgiven. Most of us naïvely believe that if someone is in love and happy they won't be tempted to have sex with anyone else. Not true. Many men, and women, attest to loving their partners dearly even though they have indulged in sex on the side. Lots don't turn down the opportunity simply because monogamy doesn't supply the electric charge and erotic high that sampling new flesh delivers. The urge to cheat exists on some level in all of us. Who gives into it and who resists it depends very much on our personal morals and relationship history. If she's able to separate sex from love – and plenty of people can – it's her way of keeping herself sexually satisfied. She's cheated on every person she's ever been out with and been forgiven for doing it, so why should she stop? It might cause you problems, but it works for her. If nothing's changed in her life to make her rethink their behaviour, it's practically guaranteed she'll repeat it. The problem with giving second chances is this: once you forgive bad behaviour, you effectively condone it. It's particularly pointless trusting her again if you knew she had a history of cheating on partners and you'd warned her you'd leave if she did it to you. If she doesn't have a history of cheating, it's early on in the relationship and this was a one-off incident with seemingly genuine reasons to explain it, hang in there, but only if she appears to be more upset about the betrayal than you are.

How long is a good period of time to have intercourse? I thought the longer the better but my new girlfriend tells me it can get boring.

Premature ejaculation is up there on most teenage boys' lists of Things I Most Fear Will Happen to Me When I Grow Up, so it's hardly surprising that many men assume the *opposite* behaviour, thrusting away for hours at a time, thinking it's a good thing. It's not. While there are some women who enjoy uninterrupted, prolonged intercourse, the majority don't. Our natural vaginal lubrication tends to dry up over a long period of time and sex becomes painful, not to mention boring. Keep on banging away in the same position for too long and we'll have mentally rehearsed the next day's work presentation five times over,

> **Brits spend an average of six days a year in bed having sex (a total of 153 hours) and nine days (211 hours) lying in bed thinking.**

rather than be panting ecstatically. It's impossible to generalize, but a quick unofficial survey came up with five to ten minutes as the preferred duration for intercourse. Most men orgasm after two minutes.

In a bid to spice things up a little I asked my husband to insert a cucumber inside me. It seemed erotic at the time but now he seems a bit huffy about it.

Men often react the same way to dildos, or anything that's remotely penis-shaped. The thing is, he's heard all the jokes about women swapping the flesh-and-blood version for a substitute because they're a lot less trouble and don't shove crisp packets down the side of the sofa, so you need to reassure him about this. You could also point out that by suggesting something sort of kinky you're displaying a healthy sexual curiosity, active imagination and willingness to share, which augers well for a varied, lusty sexual future. Oh, and if you do it again, make sure you wash the cucumber first. All those pesticides . . .

I'm struggling to cope with my husband's strange fetishes. Every time I do the washing-up with my rubber

gloves on he wants sex instantly. He also insists I masturbate him wearing them. I feel uncomfortable doing it, should I tell him?

I'm of the opinion that there's nothing wrong with indulging quirky, amusing turn-ons like this, but only if it doesn't turn into a must-have for all sex sessions and, more importantly, both of you are happy with it. You're not, which means you absolutely must talk to him about it – just make sure it's not in a judgemental way. His erotic attachment to Marigolds can probably be traced back to an event in childhood that caused him to link sexual thoughts with women washing up. One of his friends may have had a mum who was a sexy version of Bree from *Desperate Housewives*, setting off subconscious fantasies while he watched her do the housework. Let him know you're happy to indulge him now and then, but not on a frequent basis.

What's a fetish and how do I know if my partner's got one?

A fetish is an inanimate object or part of the body that turns you on. A true fetishist *must* have the thing/body part in order to be aroused and sexually satisfied. Your boyfriend asking you to parade naked in high heels for a visual treat doesn't mean he's got one. Making you wear them each and every time you have sex and not being interested otherwise suggests he does. The problem with having a fetish is that it's extremely restrictive. High heels, for instance, aren't fabulous for sex on that new sofa or velvet bedspread, and they have a habit of inserting themselves in ears, noses and eyes if you're wearing them while attempting a *Kama Sutra*-inspired position. On a more serious note, if you're worried you or your partner might have a fetish and it's interfering with your relationship, book in to see a sex therapist.

When's the right time to move in after a break-up?

This depends on how long they'd been together, how painful the break-up was, whether they emotionally left the relationship before physically leaving it and whether you're after a hot fling or a long-term liaison. If it's just sex you're after and you're being cold-hearted about it, move in while their wounds are still fresh. Splitting up from someone nearly always leaves us feeling vulnerable and we all know the quickest way to superficially boost self-esteem is to be chatted up and devoured by someone new and delicious. But of course you're far too nice to take advantage of someone, so I'll assume you want more.

As well as all of the above considerations, it depends on whether the person is male or female. Women tend to allow a grieving period when a relationship ends, rather sensibly sobbing on friends' shoulders and dissecting what went wrong. This ensures they've worked things through so they are ready for their next serious relationship with minimal baggage. Men, on the other hand, often move straight from one partner to another. I'm generalizing, but they tend not to be as good at sorting out emotional issues and often break it down to this simple equation: Have lost girlfriend/wife, need new one. Given the shortage of men, it doesn't take long (like two days) before an interested female is muscling her way in. Sure, she may be attaching herself to an emotional wreck, but she might be willing to work through his past issues to cement their future. I learned this the hard way. A man I'd adored from afar broke up with his wife and I allowed a few months to pass before calling to ask if he wanted to go for a drink. Much to my surprise, a girl answered the phone: his new live-in lover. So much for giving people time to heal!

How do I thrust when I'm on top?

This sounds like a silly question but it's not: most of the time it's him on top, so women have much less experience of it. There are two ways to position yourself, so experiment to find out which one suits you. First try squatting over him so your feet are flat – if there's a bedhead, you could lean forward and grab this for balance – and use your calf and upper thigh muscles to lift you up and down. Or straddle him so you're resting on your knees and use your upper thigh and buttock muscles to thrust. If you really can't get the hang of it, the cheat's way is to get him to hold you around the waist and lift you up and down or you stay completely still as he thrusts underneath you.

I've been with my partner for six weeks and we're having great sex, but he's suggesting we do things which are quite adventurous, and while I'm happy to try them, I'd rather wait a bit. Am I being silly?

No. While sex at the start of a relationship is typically lust-driven and enthusiastic (if it's not, move on while you have the chance) you're wise to wait until you know the person better. First up, you need to trust him in order to try adventurous (i.e. kinky things) and trust comes with time. After all, we don't want to find videos of you on the net, do we? All courtesy of that hidden camera he had installed. Secondly, the newness of the relationship should be enough of an aphrodisiac at this stage. A good time to start upping the ante is when the love hormones start to wear off and that shouldn't happen for at least another few months. When it does, you now know you're both open to trying new things, which means your sex life will stay feisty and fabulous.

I find I often get distracted during sex and start thinking about things which are totally unrelated. It's not that I'm not enjoying it, I just drift off.

If you're like most people and lead a hectic life with lots of balls in the air, this is normal, though not ideal obviously.

Being in the moment and concentrating on the sensations you're feeling during sex ups your enjoyment considerably. Try spending time winding down a little before having sex – diving into bed after rushing up stairs having just turned off your laptop/done the dishes/taken the dog for a pee isn't going to inspire you to lose yourself. Also, try keeping your eyes open rather than closed – that's to watch the action, not ponder what colour to repaint the room. Another good way to focus is to talk to your partner during lovemaking and tell him how good everything feels.

How important is love for good sex?

It's interesting. You can have magnificent sex with someone you don't love or even like that much, but just because you love someone doesn't mean the sex is going to be great. People think they go together like bacon and eggs but they don't. The ingredients for a great love affair and great sex are different. For great sex, you need bucketloads of chemistry, matching libidos, a thirst for adventure and an open mind. To love someone you need to connect on deeper emotional levels, be intellectually compatible and morally similar. This is why you might have ridiculously extraordinary orgasms with the guy who cleans the pool but disappointingly diluted ones with a husband you love dearly. The thing is, though, while your bits might sing, your heart won't.

> **Physically attractive couples are 26 per cent more likely to produce daughters than sons.**

Can using a vibrator ruin you for sex without it?

A vibrator is by far the quickest and most effective way to make a woman orgasm. Which is why they can get a teensy bit addictive when you first use one. Because it only takes mere minutes with a mechanical device, you tend to detour to the bedroom every time you make a cup of coffee (which can be a problem if you're an eight-cup-a-day girl). If you're using a vibrator this often you can temporarily numb and desensitise your genitals – meaning if your partner tries to stimulate you, you won't feel much at all. Mind you, if you're having eight orgasms a day, I'm surprised you've got the time or energy to meet up, let alone take it further.

Like most new toys, the thrill soon wears off, and before you know it you'll be down to one – OK, maybe two – DIY orgasms a day max. The only way this could now have an adverse affect on your sex life is if you train your brain to only orgasm with this type of stimulation. If all your orgasms are achieved through vibration, your brain starts to tread the same neural pathway over and over, and eventually, it starts to think this is the *only* way to orgasm and gets confused if fingers, a tongue or a penis try to accomplish the same thing (imposters!). Mix up vibrator orgasms with orgasms via stimulation with fingers, oral sex (and, if you're one of the lucky ones, penetration) and I can guarantee you won't be ruined. Spoiled maybe, but not ruined.

After years of making the effort sexually and getting rejected, I have now given up on my husband. His idea of initiating sex is to bluntly ask if I fancy it. He says he's happy with our sex life – once every ten weeks – but I say it isn't a sex life. What do I do now?

I went out with someone who also expected me to do all the work. I initiated sex, came up with new things to try and worked hard to make it special. After two years I, like you, got fed up and told him it was time for him to take over as 'sex planner'. He never did and, without nurturing, our sex life slid despondently and determinedly downhill. His laziness translated to the whole relationship, not just to sex, and I fear this is the case here.

Sit down with your husband and explain, without anger, just how unhappy you are. Then, and this is crucial, give him a blueprint of exactly what he needs to do to make you happy: how you'd like him to initiate sex and what you'd like more and less of once you're having sex. It could be that he doesn't know where to start and is too proud to ask for direction. Or it could be that he expects you to do all the work. Start with a positive slant and go from there – perhaps literally.

How hard is a penis supposed to get? My erection is never rock hard though I have normal orgasms.
There's a plethora of reasons why your erection's not Hollywood-hero hard (would James Bond ever only be semi-erect?). Physical factors include your age, how tired you are, what medication you're on, whether you've had too much to drink or indulged in drugs and how recently you've had sex. Then there are emotional influences like stress and perform-ance anxiety (I bet you haven't lost a wink of sleep worrying about this, have you? Course not.). The fact is, erections are as fickle and individual as their owners. Some mens' penises are so hard you could hammer nails with them, while others could find themselves flying at half-mast when they finally bed the woman of their dreams. The rest hover somewhere in between – sort of where you are really.

My new partner shaves his testicles and trims his pubic hair so there's hardly any down there. I got quite a shock at first – is this normal?
It depends on the man and his idea of personal grooming. While it's unusual for a woman *not* to do something to her pubic hair – we're always shaving or waxing, sometimes a little over-enthusiastically into silly heart-shapes – lots of men still consider it unmanly to do anything but give it the odd trim if things are really getting out of hand. To lots of younger guys

though, this is part of their normal grooming regime, and along with waxing chest or back hair, they'll trim and shave their pubic hair as a matter of course. An added incentive is that it makes their penises look larger. If you don't like the look, playfully suggest he lets the hair grow back because the natural look turns you on.

Does oral sex feel better if you shave off your pubic hair? My partner wants me to shave and this is his way of talking me into it.

He's right in that it allows for more skin-to-tongue contact and stops hair getting in the way (and in his mouth). But the real appeal is that, once shaved, you're far more exposed to him, and since most men are visually orientated, this is a big plus. As far as sex requests go, it's relatively painless to give this one a go, though it does itch like mad when it's growing back. If you're feeling particularly generous, work it into sex play. Hand him a razor, some shaving cream and get him to do it for you.

I'm recently divorced and new on the singles scene. I'm aware that things have changed in ten years, but a friend told me I'm supposed to put a condom on a guy before giving him oral sex. Is this true?

When the HIV hype was at its fiercest, we were all told to use dental dams (little sheets of latex) or condoms during oral sex. Viruses and infections aren't just passed on during intercourse and it makes sense to protect yourself completely if someone's sexual history isn't known to you (is it ever?). Sensible as it might be, however, using condoms for oral sex hasn't become standard sexual practice, even though it's the only way to be truly safe. Your friend is right in that it's prudent, but it's not common. Despite this, defy the norm: choose unlubricated condoms – the pre-lubed ones taste awful – or try a flavoured one; lots of brands do them.

I'm having an affair and, ironically, sex with my husband has never been better. It's confusing me. I was all set to leave, but now I'm not sure.

Just because the sex has improved doesn't mean the relationship has. It's extremely common for sex with a spouse to get better during an affair. Affair sex sends your desire levels sky high because sex becomes associated with danger and excitement, both of which are erotic uppers. Because you can't see your lover constantly there's a surplus of sexual energy, which is now directed at your husband. Add a dollop of guilt for cheating and that's why the *frisson* is back.

❶ *Women use 20,000 words a day, men use 7,000.*

Either way, I'm not surprised you're confused. It's impossible to think clearly about ending a marriage while having an affair. If you really want to make a logical, clearly-thought-through decision end it or put the affair on hold while you make up your mind.

Early menopause runs in my family and I'm terrified it will have an effect on my sex life.

The bad news is, without intervention it probably will. There are changes to pelvic and sexual organs, such as vaginal dryness, atrophy and bladder disturbances (wanting to pee or a burning sensation when you do). Then you've got mood swings, irritability, depression, hot flushes and night sweats. Not exactly a turn-on, is it? The good news is HRT (hormone replacement therapy) alleviates most of these symptoms. There are also herbal alternatives, and new research could turn up many more ways of dealing with it. By using lubricant, continuing to have sex (to keep your organs toned and libido constant) and keeping an eye on new developments, there's every chance you'll emerge from it feeling sexy and confident.

You always say to try new things sexually but when I came home with several sex books, my partner took it as a complete insult. Why?

I suspect you eagerly showed him the sex books saying he, or both of you, might learn something from them. Big mistake. Since he was a child he's been told by society that a man knows what to do in bed. To challenge this is emasculating. Don't ever quote directly from the books or an 'expert', especially not during or immediately after sex, and don't leave the books in the bedroom. A good approach is to say you bought the books because you love having sex with him and want to get a few ideas to make sure you never get bored with each other. Then casually leave them lying around because he's *so* going to sneak a peek the next time you're out.

When I orgasm I get quite dizzy, like the room is spinning, and I feel nauseous. A friend of mine says she gets headaches. Is this normal?

An orgasm is simply the release of the blood that's been pumped furiously into your genital area during arousal back into your system. In the same way as getting up too quickly can make you feel dizzy, an orgasm can make you feel the same. Wobbly legs and even a slight headache aren't unheard of, but spinning rooms and nausea? Get yourself off to see a doctor. I doubt it's anything serious but you should still check it out. Not only for health reasons but because you don't want to get into a cycle where your brain expects to feel ill after sex. Brains are sneaky and liable to stop triggering the desire for sex it if results in pain. As for your friend who gets headaches: research suggests it's more likely to happen after quick sex than a longer session, because the blood-pressure spike is more pronounced and this is usually what's responsible for the headache. If she lets herself get aroused slowly, it may solve the problem. But if it's happening regularly I'd very much like her to trot along to see a doctor with you. She's meant to get a (fake) headache *before* sex, remember?

Since my daughter was born I've gone off sex altogether. I still enjoy cuddling but when my partner tries to take it further, I panic and end up pushing him away. I can tell he's getting frustrated with me, although he'd never say anything.

It sounds like you're having difficulty merging roles. Once you became a mum you stopped being a lover: the urge to be maternal has eclipsed the urge to be sexual. In short, you've lost your sexual self. To find her again, you need several things: time (so make sure you're getting plenty of help), sleep (ditto) and to be happy out of bed (are your emotional needs being met?). Keep a sex diary: write down any erotic thoughts and what triggers them so you know what turns you on. Sort out a code word or gesture that lets you both know what's a non-sexual, affectionate cuddle and what's a come-on. Connect on sensual levels – a bubble bath together or massages – and if you're really not interested in being pleasured yourself, consider giving him oral sex, masturbating him or let him do it in front of you. Above all, give it time – it's confusing and exhausting when you first have a baby. Your desire will come back, so stop panicking and just muddle through this period as best you can. (My previous book, *Hot Relationships*, dealt with this in much more detail.)

My husband and I are both in our fifties and our children have grown up and fled the nest. We still love each other but somewhere along the line we stopped having sex. I like to think we'd outgrown that kind of thing, but my husband has started making sexual advances again recently. I've been trying to laugh it off, but frankly I find

the whole idea of sex at our age embarrassing and a little disgusting. I just can't go through with it.

Excuse me? Are you honestly saying you're too old for sex in your fifties? I've never heard anything so ridiculous in my life! I'm forty-four, six years off turning fifty, and quite frankly my sex drive is going up not down. I know *eighty*-year-olds who have a healthy sex life. It might not include all the elements their sex life did when they were twenty, but they're still clocking up plenty of orgasms and certainly doing more than saying, 'Night,' and turning over to face the wall.

Your husband is brave to finally attempt to break the sex drought and I give him full marks. He quite rightly figures it's now or never: you've done all the hard work bringing up the kids, now it's your time to enjoy yourself, and what better way to have fun than to have sex. Think back to when you were younger and recall the best sex you ever had. What did it involve? What did you used to like? Talk to your husband. Tell him you feel a bit weird and embarrassed and that you need his help to get over it. Then start by doing sexy things which don't involve sex. Start snuggling up on the sofa rather than sitting on different seats; get him to massage your shoulders; reintroduce kissing. If you feel shy, have sex with the lights off and under the covers. Do whatever it takes to get you through that first time, because I swear after you've done it once or twice, you'll wonder why you went without it all those years.

If you've never enjoyed sex, that's a different story. In that case, you might want to take yourself off for a few sessions with a sex therapist or try some of the exercises on page 206. Plenty of people say sex in their later years is the best they've had. There's a brilliant book called *Better than Ever* written by Bernie Zilbergeld which deals with sex for people post forty. Get your hands on a copy, then on your husband.

My girlfriend is more experienced than me and is always asking what I'd like more of in bed. I don't know, but I feel pressure to come up with something.

When she asks you again, whisper in her ear, 'I don't know . . . what's on offer?' That puts the ball back in her court to come up with some saucy suggestions. Another option is to flick through a good sex book – there are tons of good ideas in this one, for starters – and see what appeals. Even better, 'fess up that you haven't actually got up to that much in bed and would love her to teach you.

Are there certain things in a relationship one should never say?

Plenty. There are lots of things that, once out of our mouths, cannot be unsaid, and no amount of back-tracking, justifying or explaining is going to alter the fact that your relationship has been changed forever because of it. The really bad things ('I don't love you and never have') we tend to shout in arguments; others ('Your bum looks big in *everything* so yes, it looks big in that too!') come tumbling out in moments of intense irritation. Either way, damage is done, and sometimes it's irreparable. I am all for honesty in relationships, but I do not, never have and never will condone the nothing-should-be-secret rule some couples insist on. There's honesty and there's stupidity. Honesty is sitting down with your partner and saying 'You know what? I think we should try something new this weekend. Jazz things up a bit in the bedroom.' Stupidity is saying, 'I am a heartbeat away from sleeping with someone at work because I'm bored silly with our sex life.' Stupidity is answering, 'Is my best friend prettier than me?' with, 'Sorry, honey, but yes she is.' Sensitivity is saying, 'Look, she's pretty – there's no denying that – but she's nowhere near as sexy as you and she's not my type.'

Assuming you don't intend to act on it, telling your

partner you fancy one of their friends or workmates accomplishes nothing but hurts the person you supposedly love and stirs up unnecessary jealousy. Ditto telling your partner you loved an ex more than them or had better sex with someone else. Comparing your partner unfavourably to others, physically, intellectually or emotionally, isn't terribly helpful in any circumstance, and putting them down in front of friends or family is unforgiveable. I also don't condone confessing about affairs or one-night stands you now consider a horrible mistake, unless they are about to find out anyway. *You* did it, *you* live with the guilt. Confessing destroys trust and often the relationship at the expense of having no secrets. Plenty of people wish their partner had never told them about an indiscretion. Says one battle-scarred male friend: 'I figured not too many people stay married for more than twenty years without being tempted now and then. Intellectually I could live with that, what I couldn't live with was my partner confirming it had happened and providing details. If she hadn't told me, we'd still be happy together. Now our whole marriage is over because of one stupid lapse of judgement.' Think before you speak.

> **It really is better to have loved and lost than never to have loved at all. In a survey of almost 70,000 Americans, US professors found people who never married die earlier than those who are divorced, separated or widowed.**

My previous boyfriend used to constantly make fun of the face I make when I orgasm. It's made me really self-conscious and I'm now dreading having sex with any future boyfriends.

He's obviously an ex for a reason: tactlessness. Lots of us make weird orgasm faces, and I have to say, the more passionate the lover, the weirder the face. So he should take it as a compliment. Good sex is sloppy, sweaty and immensely unflattering. We hyperventilate, frown, scream, show our tonsils and do a lot of scrunching up of our faces. You're normal. I suspect the teasing was prompted by jealousy: he wished *he* could lose himself in the moment so totally.

Is it time to stop looking and settle for what I can get?
'Settling' – deciding you're not going to get the type of partner you'd hoped for, so settling for second, third or fourth best – is an interesting concept. If you've been actively looking for your ideal match the whole of your life, you're now eighty-five and haven't met anyone yet, 'settling' is probably prudent. If you're twenty-five and foaming at the mouth because everyone else is getting married, it's not. I have to admit, the whole concept of settling turns my (and maybe your) stomach because I would rather be single and enjoying my friends than with someone I didn't honestly admire, respect or fancy. But that's me. I've got lots of single friends to play with, which means single is fun not lonely, tend to go on lots of dates and meet lots of new people all the time. So there's still that feeling that Mr Ideal might pop up at any moment. When all my friends are couples and I stop being asked out, I suspect I might feel very differently. Some good questions to ask yourself if you're considering it are: is my 'ideal' partner a figment of my imagination? In other words, does the person you are waiting for exist or do you need to make your must-haves a little more realistic? Are you female and do you want children? If you're approaching forty and being super fussy, this might alter your selection process. How often do you meet single, eligible people? If it's once every ten years, I'd be looking damn hard at the next one. Finally, what's more important to you: chemistry, soul-mate connection and an intense emotional bond or

compatibility, companionship and a respect for the institution of marriage? If it's the former, settling for anything less probably won't make you happy anyway; if it's the latter it probably will.

I sometimes find myself having sex just to be polite. It seems easier and less fuss to do it rather than try to get out of it if I've changed my mind. Is this normal?
It depends on the situation. If you mean agreeing to sex after one date that didn't go well, no it's not normal. That's passively giving the nod to date rape and having zero respect for sex, yourself and your body. If, however, you mean you've been seeing someone for a bit and you've got yourself in a situation where sex is very much on the agenda, but somewhere between planning it and enthusiastically agreeing to the sexy night in/weekend away/holiday, you changed your mind, I get where you're coming from. A quick ring around turned up three female friends who'd definitely gone along with sex in this situation: 'I didn't want to hurt him', 'It seemed rude when we'd been seeing each other for weeks and it was obvious it was expected', 'I really fancied him but then when I saw his penis, I didn't. It would have been really obvious to stop at that point and I didn't want to give him a complex'. Five male friends admitted to 'polite sex' as well: 'I didn't find her attractive naked but knew she'd be upset so I pretended to fancy her', 'My ex had called that day and I knew we'd get back together but it seemed rude not to have sex when we'd already planned to'. Nearly *all* my male friends admitted to having sex when they really didn't feel like it and/or fancy the girl simply because it's an opportunity to have sex. See how far we've all progressed? (Not.)

I'm not saying I haven't done the same thing – I have – but having sex just to be polite isn't ideal. I mean how difficult can it be to say, 'Look, I'm really sorry about this but it isn't working out for me and I think I'd like us just to be friends'? Come on, you're not sixteen any more, you're a grown-up! And if you are sixteen, all the more reason to say no! It might be time to steel yourself for a few disappointed faces than let someone have their way when you really don't want them to.

I've just found out my husband had an affair. We are planning on getting counselling immediately but I'm not sure if it's best to go together or separately.

It depends on the couple and the style of counselling, but I'd advise having at least a few sessions each solo, as well as lots together. I know several psychologists who specialize in post-infidelity cases and they say the two sexes tend to work through the fall-out in different ways. Men who've had affairs tend to look forward and don't want to relive it all again. Women who've been cheated on want to look back in order to revisit and understand what happened. As well as this, both sexes sometimes have issues over leaving their lover, which the innocent partner shouldn't have to endure, such as guilt over saying goodbye and mourning their loss. Hearing things like this is incredibly hurtful and should be dealt with privately.

I didn't have a huge sex drive before I got pregnant, but now that's all I can think about. Why?

In a word: hormones. Your body has such a high concentration of female and pregnancy hormones that your breasts and sex organs are more sensitive and responsive than they have ever been, and perhaps ever will be, which is something positive to focus on when your partner excitedly suggests you have another baby only minutes after what felt like a 300-year labour! Plenty of pregnant women find sex more exciting and satisfying during this period – many experience orgasm for the first time while others have multiples. A rise of oestrogen causes an increase in blood flow to the pelvic area, which in turn causes stretching and swelling, which normally only happens when you're sexually excited. This means your sensory nerve endings are hypersensitive without any stimulation at all, which means *rapid* arousal. Your breasts are bigger – a turn on for both of you if you never progressed past a training bra – and pregnancy also causes you to secrete more vaginal fluid, so you feel and are ready for penetration earlier. It's entirely safe, by the way, to have sex whenever you want to, so long as it's not too athletic and you haven't been advised not to for medical reasons. Conception and pregnancy guru, Dr Miriam Stoppard, says it's actually safe to have intercourse right up till the point when you go into labour. I can't imagine too many women taking advantage of this, but it's certainly an alternative to flicking through piles of old magazines.

 FOR HER

SEX SOLUTIONS TO SUIT EVERY SCENARIO

Too tired, too bloated, too drunk? Beat the lust-busters with a move for every moment and mood.

1. You're having a fat day

What you want: A position which hides bulges and keeps you semi-covered, and preferably stops his hands going anywhere near your tummy, love handles or other current no-go zones.

Intimate instructions: We all know sex is about what's happening on the inside not the outside, but let's face it, no-one feels like parading in suspenders on a truly bad body day. There are alternatives to keeping your T-shirt on and settling for (yawn) missionary though. Rear-entry positions are the most flattering for most bods. Kneel facing away from him, lean down to rest your weight on your forearms and push your bottom tantalizingly high in the air, in his direction. Not only does it give him a visual treat, the angle and position makes your waist look tiny and your thighs slim and taut. It cleverly and effectively hides your other bits because you're leaning forward out of view, and all without you having to launch into that whiny, 'Don't look at my tummy,' girly stuff. Get him to put his hands on your hips to hold you steady while he thrusts and you've also solved the wandering hands problem. If you're really self-conscious, lean forward onto a pile of pillows to cover your tummy.

A new angle: If you do opt for missionary, make a podgy upper midriff look sexier by stretching your arms up over your head and grabbing onto the bedposts. If there aren't any, twist your palms and place them flat on the wall behind the bed. Better still, grab his hands and get him to pin you there. It's supersexy for him because he's in control and you're completely submissive, and it works a treat for making tummies look flat and breasts perky.

2. You're half-asleep

What you want: A zero-effort session where he won't notice if you nod off during the boring bits, plus a super-speedy orgasm for him so you can be snoring in the spoon position in no time.

Intimate instructions: Chances are you're lying in this position anyway, eyes determinedly shut, despite his penis prodding you in the back, so this really is lazy-girl sex. You're on your side, your back to his front, now lift your bottom to allow him to penetrate, then tighten your thighs for maximum friction. His hands can then reach around to stimulate your clitoris – you might want it over and done with, but that shouldn't stop you sneaking in a quick orgasm as well. To speed him up, make lots of satisfied groans and moans.

A new angle: If you can bear to get out of bed or are already snuggled up in front of the telly, have armchair sex instead. You sit on his lap, facing him, in a crouched position. Place your feet flat on the seat beside his thighs or on the chair arms, he holds you by the waist and lifts you up and down. If you really want to be self-indulgent, tell him it's 'your turn' sex and he'll get to be completely spoilt next time. Settle yourself in that swivel chair in the study for a blissful oral sex session and solve any height differences by letting him use the controls to move you into the perfect position.

3. You've got your period

What you want: A position which doesn't bump or show off a bloated, tender tummy, and doesn't involve washing the sheets afterward. Ironically, while some women want nothing more than bed and a hot water bottle, lots of women are turned on more during their period than at any other time of the month. Here's another incentive to get over any squeamishness: an orgasm often cures period pain.

Intimate instructions: The shower is an obvious choice given the mess problem, but it works for other reasons: warm water running over your abdomen feels soothing if you've got period bloat. Face away from the water. It may look marvellously sexy letting water stream over your cheekbones (not to mention brave since your make-up will be disappearing down the drain) but you move your head more than you think during sex and water shooting up your nose *isn't* so hot. How this works depends a little on your height differences. Try putting your hands on the shower wall for balance, and let him enter from behind as you stand on tip-toes and push your bottom up and outward. Alternatively, put your back against the shower wall and lift one leg as high as you can, resting your calf against the side of his shoulder. He holds your thigh and under your bottom to support you. By choosing a position where you're in charge of the pace, rhythm and depth of penetration – him behind or you on top – sensitive cervixes and sore tummies can be catered for. Another good option which saves the bedclothes: do it in the kitchen. Those easy-clean surfaces are there for a reason. You hop on the counter, while he stands in front and penetrates, you either wrap your legs around his waist or put them on chairs or stools to give leverage and stability. Be warned, though, the angle is deep. It'll either hurt a little (in which case, tilt your bottom back to keep thrusting shallow) or he'll hit your G-spot, which you possibly won't complain about.

A new angle: If it seemed like a great idea but thrusting starts to hurt, get him to withdraw and use the head of his penis to rub against your clitoris until you orgasm, then finish him off with your hand or mouth.

4. You're taking ages to orgasm

What you want: An orgasm . . . now! As much as it feels exquisite hovering at that lovely I-think-I'm-about-to-but-then-again-maybe-not stage, getting stuck there isn't as much fun.

Intimate instructions: The trick is to switch stimulation – you've probably desensitised yourself by doing the same thing for so long your body needs a kick to push it over the edge. Try adding something new. If you're into anal stimulation, a well-lubricated finger delivered with sensitivity and timing could do the trick. If that's not your cup of tea, try the old fake-it-till-you-make-it method. *Pretend* you're going into the throes of orgasm – clench your bottom and thighs, moan and throw your head back – and you may trick your body into doing just that by providing all the triggers it associates with orgasm. Didn't work? Then change position. Get him to lie on his back, legs stretched out and together, then climb on top so you have complete control. Put your knees on either side of his chest, let him penetrate and, leaning forward, move your hips in small circles so your clitoris makes contact with his pubic bone. It's also easy to climb off from here and move yourself upwards: if his penis isn't doing it for you, his tongue might.

A new angle: Make it a threesome by reaching down, opening your bedside drawer and getting out your vibrator. Switch to a rear-entry position while one of you holds the vibrator firmly on the fleshy bit directly above the clitoris.

5. You've both had too much to drink

What you want: A way to make the most of your alcohol-induced lack of inhibition without landing you both in jail. Help with a wonky erection wouldn't go astray either.

Intimate instructions: The second you're in the front door – better still, don't shut it completely – go for it! Don't remove your clothes, just unzip and pull your panties to one side – having sex while fully clothed feels lustily risqué, as if you just can't wait. Let him slam you up against the hallway wall, you stand with legs spread, then lift one and turn it sideways so he can penetrate. He puts his hand under your thigh for support, you put your arms around his neck for balance. Another way to be naughty but not risk anything is to do it in front of a window with the lights off. You can see everyone else walking past/watching telly, so it feels like you're wantonly having sex in front of them, but they can't see you.

A new angle: If you can feel his erection draining, get him in a position where he's on top. Gravity then works in his favour, keeping all the blood in the penis rather than draining out of it. Don't panic if he's too limp for intercourse and resist the urge to dive down and desperately perform the kiss of life. This could work or it could make him even more paranoid. I'd avoid his penis entirely until he seems relaxed, sneaking a peek occasionally to see if anything's happening. Tell him you don't need an erect penis to have a good time in bed, his tongue and fingers will do just fine, thank you.

WHAT ARE THE LATEST, GREATEST SEX TOYS AND HOW DO I CHOOSE AND USE THEM?

One of the quickest ways to introduce novelty in your sex life is to invite a nice, new, shiny, probably pink plaything into it. This is one threesome I heartily approve of: you, your partner and a sex toy (or two or three). The reason why sex toys loom large on spice-up-your-sex-life lists is because a) as the name suggests, they're fun and b) if it vibrates, she's instantly light years ahead in the probability-of-an-orgasm race. Despite glowing reports from users, however, few people stroll nonchalantly into a sex store on the high street. Instead, we tap away excitedly at home online and end up . . . confused. There's an alarming array of goods out there to choose from, and given that you can't actually pick them up and examine them properly, it's hard to know where to start. To help you along, I've compiled a list of the most likely items you'll click on and recommended some websites. Rest assured, by the way, almost all purchases arrive in brown packaging *minus* a sticker saying '10-inch throbbing dildo inside' (check out the site's packaging policy if you're at all worried). I do a sex-toy range which you can access via my websites **www.traceycoxshop.com** or **www.traceycoxshopusa.com**, other reputable places to try include **www.lovehoney.co.uk**, **www.passiononline.co.uk** or **www.sh-womenstore.com**, **www.goodvibes.com**, **www.mypleasure.com** and **www.xandria.com**. If you're going to splash some cash, here's a guide to what does and *doesn't* do what it says on the box.

Vibrators: There's everything from a rubber duck to something that looks like it should be in a cage. Narrow your choice by thinking about your individual needs. Do you want penetration? If so, the infamous 'rabbit' – a penis-shaped vibrator with a clitoral attachment – is a good choice. If you decide you don't fancy penetration, turn it around and simply use the clitoral stimulator. The most versatile in terms of size and all-round use is probably a 'wand' vibrator. It's a compact, cylindrical vibrator which you hold against the clitoris while masturbating or during intercourse. It's an almost guaranteed way for women to orgasm during penetration and because it's not big or sculpted to look like a penis (no veins, promise) it's non-threatening for him.

Searching for a strong vibration? Opt for one that looks like a back massager – large with a large rounded head – like the Hitachi Magic Wand, which plugs into a main power supply rather than relying on batteries. Don't worry, they are 100 per cent safe. As a general rule, if the vibrator is made of hard plastic it will hold the vibration better. Rubber or silicone feel and look nice, but they're usually weaker. Gadget vibrators – remote controls, lipsticks, mobile phones, you name it, they've got it – make fun presents, but steer clear if you're only making one purchase. You'll also find lots of vibrators designed to particularly target your G-spot or front vaginal wall. Lots of people swear they're the best invention since, well, the original vibrator. Other factors to consider are variable speeds, quietness and whether it's waterproof.

Dildos: If vibrators didn't exist, these would be far more popular. Given that they're basically penises of varying sizes and they don't vibrate, a lot of women are like 'Huh? Why would I want one of those if I can't orgasm through penetration anyway?' The answer is that they're good for fantasy or role-play, some women like to feel 'full' during oral sex, some men like to be penetrated anally (though there are toys designed expressly for this purpose) and they're obviously handy for lesbians who like penetration. Some are S shaped for G-spot stimulation. If you want to strap one on, you'll also need a harness, which attaches it to you via straps around your thighs and bottom. Some harnesses have a second dildo which fits inside the vagina or anus.

Love balls: The original version are called Ben Wa Balls – two separate small balls which you insert into your vagina while simply going about your business – popping out for a sandwich at lunch, for instance. Why this is supposed to put a spring in your step, rather than a bizarre limp, is perplexing since most women don't orgasm through penetration alone. I'd give them a miss if I were you. You'll also find duo-tone vibe balls. These are small connected balls which vibrate. They're designed for G-spot stimulation, but are also quite good for pelvic floor toning if you squeeze your muscles around them repetitively. These score extra points because at least they vibrate, but they're still not my favourite sex toy.

Pelvic floor toners: The more toned her vaginal muscles, the better sex will be for both of you since she'll be able to grip his penis tighter. You can rhythmically squeeze the muscles, doing sets on a repetitive basis (called Kegel exercises) without inserting one of these gadgets. But having something to grip onto means you're more likely to be doing the exercises correctly. Most of them resemble tiny barbells which work on weight resistance. Highly recommended after childbirth but handy for anyone who wants to keep *all* their parts in shape.

Penis rings: These are rings made of rubber, leather or metal which men slip onto a flaccid or semi-erect penis. Because the

Female and want to stay interested in sex? Don't commit to a long-term relationship. German researchers found that four years into a relationship, less than half of thirty-year-old women want regular sex while the man's libido stayed the same!

ring is tight, it traps blood in the penis, helping maintain a stronger erection for longer. Men who are a little on the (ahem) small side will probably like it because they make the penis look and feel bigger. The problem is, men with smaller penises tend to be premature ejaculators – not very fair I know, but it's because the penis head has roughly the same amount of nerves concentrated over a smaller surface. Since penis rings tend to increase sensitivity, he could orgasm sooner than usual. (You win some, you lose some.) If you want to try one, opt for rubber first – leather is more expensive and metal's a bit scary – but make sure it fits snugly around the penis and isn't too loose. Don't leave it on for more than twenty minutes and whatever you do, remove it before you snuggle up for the night.

Vibrating penis rings: They're penis rings, usually rubber, with little vibrators attached for clitoral stimulation. I've got one in my range, but I have to say I wasn't convinced at first. The reason why is that if you use the traditional in-out thrusting the vibrator doesn't maintain contact with the clitoris for long enough to be effective. Use a grinding, circular motion, however, with him keeping his pelvis pressed close against yours during intercourse, and you, like me, may get a *very* pleasant surprise!

Anal toys: Anal vibrators are squatter than usual, with a flared base, so what goes up doesn't stay up there! They can be used on both men and women in a variety of ways, during oral sex or by leaving them in during intercourse. Soft and jelly-like, 'butt plugs' stay in better, though they don't vibrate. Anal beads are plastic balls threaded onto a thin nylon cord and they look like something your three-year-old would present you with after a craft class. You insert them, then pull them out right before or during orgasm.

Vibrating sleeves: Vibrating sleeves are a masturbatory device which is meant to replicate the female cavity. I haven't heard great reports. You can also buy textured gloves for both male and female masturbation, which are supposed to increase sensation. Use with lube or you'll shoot through the roof for all the wrong reasons.

Whips, paddles and riding crops: All used for spanking and not as threatening as you'd first imagine. That soft rubber whip swishes through the air making a menacing sound but lands with a whisper-soft touch. All talk and no action, which is exactly what you want for role-play. Riding crops come in pretty colours but add a frown and you're transformed into a menacing mistress. Paddles – hard wooden things which look a bit like misshapen ping-pong bats – are more for serious S & M devotees. They *hurt* and it's hard to judge how hard you're hitting with one.

S & M gear: Gimp masks, dog-collars, dangerously studded-looking leather outfits – it's enough to make the timid log off pronto, suddenly deciding it's all a bad idea. If you're curious, start off with some handcuffs or a studded collar, then work your way up to full leather outfits, masks and serious bondage gear. It costs a fortune and there's no try-before-you-buy, so make sure it's not just a passing phase. Yes they'll come in awfully handy for that fancy dress ball but your friends will never look at you quite the same afterwards.

Dressing up clothes: PVC nurses' outfits, baby-doll lingerie, all-in-one catsuits – they're straight out of the eighties and tons of fun. Be warned though: you'll pay through the nose for them in a sex shop and they're not terribly well made. If you're flush and you like the look of them, though, why not?

Lingerie for her: Own more lingerie than Paris Hilton, mix it up a bit by choosing different types for different moods and you've hit on a winning formula. Team sexy 'boy shorts' with tight T-shirts, try lurid bras with nipple cut-outs and 'easy access' crotchless knickers – visit Myla or Agent Provocateur for gorgeous versions. Wear a pure white lacy bra, G-string, stockings and suspenders for 'innocent' role-plays. It'll make you feel sexier and the average highly visual male will adore it.

WHAT ARE LOVE DRUGS?

Well, they're not drugs like cocaine or Ecstasy. However fabulous *they* might feel at the time, the effect isn't quite as sexy when your nose caves in. The real love drugs are what our bodies produce naturally when we're attracted and aroused by someone. These, by the way, are every bit as powerful and addictive as the manufactured variety, just ask a 'love junkie' – someone whose relationships fizzle out fast once the hormones wear off.

Knowing what's produced when isn't just interesting to know, it can help you work through the inevitable ups and downs of nature's love rollercoaster. Is it a hormonal hiccup you're going through or are you just not suited? It could well depend on where you're at in the cycle.

Norepinephrine and dopamine: Our hormone levels of both dopamine and norepinephrine soar when we're confronted by the unknown. In the initial stage of romantic love, when everything is new, these two trigger such exhilaration we lose the desire to eat or sleep. The feelings of euphoria are created by these elevated levels, which electrify the reward system in the brain. The only way to keep this potent pair surging through our bloodstream is to either constantly change partners or to introduce as much novelty as possible into a long-term relationship, tricking the brain into pumping it out. Couples who share exciting experiences consistently report much more relationship satisfaction than those who don't. Sex is another way to rev it up as sex elevates testosterone, which in turn revs up dopamine levels.

Oxytocin: This is hormonal superglue. It's released after dopamine subsides and is designed to lead to long-term attachment. While dopamine and norepinephrine make you feel excited and edgy, oxytocin is a cuddle chemical, making you feel warm and fuzzy. Along with vasopressin, it's what bonds you as a couple, making you feel like settling down and having children. It also induces drowsiness. Oxytocin is the reason why men want to drift off to sleep straight after sex. It's released into the male bloodstream two to five minutes after orgasm and into the female bloodstream about twenty to thirty minutes afterwards. Just giving us time for us to pop down and do the dishes, then turn off the lights while he's snoring comfortably away – not.

Useful Contacts and Resources

These sources have been particularly helpful in my research:

WEBSITES
www.bettydodson.com – Masturbation workshops in the US
www.anniesprinkle.org – Classes and workshops in the US
www.nerve.com – Cool, edgy sex information and forum
www.sexualhealth.com – Sexual health information
www.netdoctor.co.uk – Good, easy-to-understand medical info
www.fpa.org.uk – The Family Planning Association UK
www.plannedparenthood.org – Contraception and Parenting
    US
www.relate.org.uk – Counselling and Sex Therapy UK
www.bps.org.uk – British Psychological Society
www.basrt.org.uk – British Association for Sexual and
    Relationship Therapy
www.psychologytoday.com – Great sex info and list of
    psychologists in the US
www.sexaa.org – Counselling for sex addicts
www.traceycox.com – General sex info and book excerpts
www.traceycoxshop.com – Sex toys and tips on using them

www.lovehoney.co.uk – Sex toys and aids
www.goodvibes.com – Sex toys and hints on how to use them

MAGAZINES

Psychology Today, published bimonthly by Sussex Publishers (US) www.psychologytoday.com

Psychologies, published bimonthly by Hachette Filpacchi (UK) www.psychologies.co.uk

READING LIST
Good general sex info:

Hot Sex: How to Do It, Tracey Cox (Corgi Books, 1998)

supersex, Tracey Cox (Dorling Kindersley, 2002)

superhotsex, Tracey Cox (Dorling Kindersley, 2002)

For Women Only, Jennifer Berman and Laura Berman (Virago, 2001)

The Big Bang, Em & Lo (Emma Taylor and Lorelei Sharkey) (Penguin, 2003)

The Sex Book, Suzi Godson, Mel Agace and Robert Winston (Cassell Illustrated, 2002)

The New Male Sexuality, Bernie Zilbergeld (Bantam Books, 1999)

Secrets of Sexual Ecstasy, Michael S. Broder and Arlene Goldman (Alpha Books, 2004)

The Sensual Touch, Dr Glenn Wilson (Caroll and Graf, 1996)

Intimate Touch, Dr Glenn Wilson (Little, Brown and Company, 1990)

The Relate Guide to Sex in Loving Relationships, Sarah Litvinoff (Vermilion, 1999)

Sex Tips for Straight Women from a Gay Man, Dan Anderson and Maggie Berman (Harper Collins, 1997)

The Magic of Sex, Dr Miriam Stoppard (Dorling Kindersley, 2001)

How to Give Her Absolute Pleasure, Lou Paget (Broadway Books, 2000)

How to Be a Great Lover, Lou Paget (Broadway Books, 1999)

She Comes First, Ian Kerner (Regan Books, 2004)

The New Good Vibrations Guide to Sex, Cathy Winks and Anne Semans (Cleis Press, 1997)

Long-term sex, mismatched libidos, low desire:

The Erotic Mind, Jack Morin (HarperCollins, 1996)

Resurrecting Sex, David Schnarch (Quill, 2002)

The Sex Starved Marriage, Michele Weiner Davis (Simon & Schuster, 2003)

I'm Not in the Mood, Judith Reichman (William Morrow, 1998)

Electrify your Sex Life, Carole Altman (Sourcebooks, 2004)

Quickies, Tracey Cox (Dorling Kindersley, 2006)

The Sex Inspector's Masterclass, Tracey Cox and Michael Alvear (Michael Joseph, 2005)

Better than Ever, Bernie Zilbergeld (Crown, 2004)

Families, past and other influences:

Families and How to Survive Them, Robin Skynner and John Cleese (Vermilion, 1997)

Sex Smart, Aline Zoldbrod (New Harbinger Publications, 1998)

Gay and Lesbian:

The Straight Girl's Guide to Sleeping with Chicks, Jen Sincero (Fireside, 2005)

Born Gay, Dr Glenn Wilson and Qazi Rahman (Peter Owen, 2004)

The Whole Lesbian Sex Book, Felice Newman (Cleis Press, 1999)

Infidelity:

NOT "Just Friends", Shirley Glass and Jean Coppock Staeheli (Simon & Schuster, 2003)

(All Shirley Glass titles are highly recommended)

Anatomy of Love, Helen Fisher (Fawcett Books, 1992)

Hot Relationships: How to Have One, Tracey Cox (Corgi Books, 1999)

Multiple orgasms, spiritual sex:

Expanded Orgasm, Patricia Taylor (Sourcebooks, 2002)

The Multi-Orgasmic Man, Mantak Chai and Douglas Abrams Arava (HarperCollins, 1997)

Find out more about Tracey by visiting www.traceycox.com or buy her books and products on www.traceycoxshop.com or www.lovehoney.co.uk

Index

A-spot, 128, 132–3
addiction to sex, 143–4
affairs *see* infidelity
age
    ejaculation and, 208–9
    enjoyment of sex and, 5, 208, 269–70
    genitals and, 197
AIDS (acquired immune deficiency syndrome), 34, 35, 104,
    232–3, 266 *see also* STIs
alcohol, 49, 92
    failure to ejaculate and, 25
    safe sex and, 232
    sensitivity and, 25, 102, 280–1
    vagina and, 207
Alvear, Michael, 246
anal fingering, 51, 101–4, 209
anal sex, 104–6
    sex toys and, 104, 233–5, 235, 284
    STIs and, 233
    trying for first time, 92, 104–5
androgen, 140
anorgasmia (inability to have an orgasm), 211
anti-depressants, 205, 208
aphrodisiacs, 135–41
Arava, Douglas, 123
ArginMax, 140
arousal systems, 47, 88, 107–11, 213–14
attractiveness, 2–7
authority figure, dreams of sex with, 146

bad beliefs, breaking free of, 67–8
bad sex, 22–5, 143–4
barrier contraception *see* condoms; contraception
BASRT, 206
Ben Wa Balls, 283
Better than Ever (Zilbergeld), 270
birth control *see* contraception
bisexuality, 223–5
    see also gay men; lesbian
blindfolding, 178
blow job *see* oral sex
body, worrying about during sex, 3–4, 10, 46–7, 51, 101, 276
body odour, male, 51
bodymap, drawing a, 63–4
books
    erotic, 92, 188, 218
    sex manuals, 19, 92, 268, 271
break-up, moving in after a, 261
breasts
    foreplay and, 12
    massaging during oral sex, 79, 82
    stimulating, 192
bridge manoeuvre, 116–17, 211
Bright, Susie, 136

calendar, erotic, 91
CAT (coital alignment technique), 211
celebrities
    dreaming of sex with, 145, 178
    influence on sex life, 60–1
cheating *see* infidelity
chemistry, how important is, 11
Chia, Mantak, 123
child abuse 212
chlamydia 34, 104
Cialis, 136–7
Cleopatra, 78
clitoris, 138, 191, 192
    bulbs, 128
    dildos and, 236

clitoris (*cont.*)
    how to find, 128–9
    oral sex and, 76–7, 79, 81
    orgasm and, 108, 115, 117, 124, 128–9, 132
    roadtest, 129
    touching, 40, 57, 103
    what is it?, 128–9
commitment, fear of, 12–13
common mistakes
    men make, 39–44
    women make, 44–8
compliments
    after sex, 12
    desire and, 162–3
    during sex, 12
condoms, 8, 15, 19, 21, 33
    breaking, 33
    dildos and, 235
    and oral sex, 266
contraception
    barrier methods, 33
        see also condoms
    Depo-Provera shot, 33
    diaphragm, 33
    emergency solutions, 32–4
    IUD, 33
    Pill, 32–3, 206
    triphasic, 140, 206
    withdrawal method, 33
contracts, 198–204, 215, 217
counselling, couples, 275
criticising your partner, 38, 73
cunnilingus *see* oral sex

delay creams, 137
Depo Provera 33
    see also contraception
desensitization techniques, 209, 249
desire
    acting upon, 216

cycle of, 87–8
as a decision, 216
early stages of relationship and, 2, 36–7
ejaculation and, 45–6, 208–10
loss of, 206
monogamy and, 2, 159–163, 172–83, 207
see also arousal systems, libido
detox, sex, 199–204
diary, sex, 206
differentiation, 180–1
dilators, 212
dildo *see* sex aids, vibrator
diseases, sexually transmitted, see STIs
dopamine, 286
dreams
    interpreting sexual, 145–6
    sharing, 186
dressing, sexy, 88, 285
    see also role play
drugs
    Cialis, 136–7
    erectile dysfunction, 135–8, 208
    for her, 138–41
    for him, 135–8
    Levitra, 137
    love, 286–7
        see also hormones
    safe, 232
    testosterone boosters, 137–8
dry humping, 34

ejaculation
    female, 134–5
    non-ejaculatory orgasm (NEO), 120, 121
    penis size and, 254–5
    premature, 19, 25, 209–10, 254–5, 258–9, 284
    retarded, 208–9
Electrify Your Sex Life (Altman), 199, 201–2
emotional intelligence, 4, 127
erectile dysfunction, 135–8, 207–8

erection, hardness of 265
Eros therapy, 139
erotic
    books 92, 188, 218
    films, 178, 223
Erotic Mind, The (Morin), 179
ex-lovers
    dreaming of sex with, 146
    influence on future sex life, 59–60
    sex with, 149–50
exercise, sexual appetite and, 216
experimentation, reactions to suggestions of, 48, 183–5, 207

family, influence of on sex life, 13–14, 61–2, 111–12, 213
fantasies 127
    celebrity, 60–1, 145
    exercises, 207
    exploring, 183–5, 206
    female, 40–1
    infidelity and, 170
    in marriage, 147
    sex with another woman, 185
    sharing, 181–9
    threesomes, 185–6
fellatio *see* oral sex
Femidom, 129
    see also contraception
fetishes, 259–60
first night/date sex, 8–9, 71
first time sex
    top five things he's hoping you'll do, 10
    top five things she's hoping you'll do, 12
fisting, 237–42
    anal, 240–2
    vaginal 237–40
foreplay, 73
    all-day, 88–93
    texting as, 90
    tips for males, 12, 42–3
    for virgins, 19–20

frenulum, 210
friends
    are you too close for sex? 178–82
    dreams of sex with, 147
front wall stimulation *see* vagina

G-shot, 140–1
G-spot, 54, 102, 125, 130–1, 132, 134, 282
gay men, 101, 241–6
    coming out to relatives, 251
    gaydar, 224–5
    hands and, 236–7
    porn, 189
    straight guys' guide to having sex with gay men, 241–6
gay women *see* lesbians
genes, libido and, 111–12, 213
genital herpes, 34, 35, 233
    see also STIs
genital warts, 34, 35, 232
    see also STIs
genitals
    age and, 173, 197
    complimenting, 82–3
    exercises, 25, 73, 125
    healthy, 173, 197
Glass, Shirley, 155, 166
Gonorrhoea 34, 35
    see also genitals, STIs
Gottman, John, 162, 192
group sex, 154, 185–6
gynaecologist
    attraction towards, 165–6
    visiting, 212

hair
    pulling during sex, 252–3
    trimming pubic, 265–6
Halban's fascia, 133–4
handjob, 98–101, 247–8
handcuffs, 187, 285

Healing Tao instructor, 123
hepatitis, 34, 35, 104, 233
    see also genitals; STIs
herpes
    genital, 35, 104, 233
        see also genitals; STIs
high heels, 58
HIV (human immunodeficiency virus), 34, 104, 233, 266
    see also STIs
Holstege, Gert, 110–11
homosexuality see gay men, lesbians
hormones
    attachment, 69, 87
    female, 40
    happy, 128
    levels, 206
    sleep inducing, 45, 87, 109, 120
Hot Relationships (Cox), 269
Hot Sex: How to Do It (Cox), 80, 211
Hotter Sex (Cox), 143
How to make love to the same person for the rest of your life – and still love it (O'Connor), 173
HPV (human papilloma virus – warts), 34, 233
    see also STIs
HRT (hormone replacement therapy), 138–9, 267

impotence, 135–6, 207–8
infidelity, 143–4
    counselling, 275
    does it matter if no one knows?, 166–7
    does sex with an ex count?, 149–50
    emotional, 168–71
    forgiving, 258
    look but don't touch, 167–71
    married people, 256–7, 267, 275
    with a sex worker, 20–1
    should I come clean about?, 157–8
    wanting to commit, 207
    why you're tempted, 156–64
    see also monogamy

instructions, women giving men, 47–8
intercourse
    changing positions during, 43, 50–1, 128, 204
    digging deep position, 52, 53
    femoral, 89
    painful, 211–12
    rear entry, 51, 54–5, 57, 117
    reverse wall thrust (standing) position, 56
    the sex squat, 52, 54–5
    sex without, 43
    sideways swoon (side entry), 55–6
    top bottom position, 51, 52–3
    woman on top, 117, 261–2
intimacy exercises, 201–2
IUD (intrauterine device) 33
    see also contraception

K-Y Jelly *see* lubricants
Kama Sutra, 143
Kegel exercises, 25, 71, 125, 212, 283
kinky sex, dreams of, 147
Kinsey, Alfred, xii, 127, 226, 231
kissing
    bad breath and, 95
    as foreplay, 89–90
    grown-ups' guide to, 94–8
    necks, 96
    penis or vagina, 95
    STIs and, 34, 233
    tongues, 95–6

lesbians 219–39
    ejaculation and, 134–5
    fantasies, 185
    finger size and, 236–7
    hasbians, 223
    porn, 189
    safe sex, 232–3
    scissoring, 233
    straight girls guide to sex with, 225–31

lesbians (*cont.*)
  vanilla, 231
  where to meet, 227
Levitra, 137
libido
  children and, 269–70
  high, 2, 23
  inherited, 61, 111–12
  loss of, 205
  low, 23, 140, 141, 205
  men's, 39–40, 45, 148
  mismatched, 207, 213–18
  pregnancy and, 275–6
  women's, 138–40, 141, 205
lists
  of favourite things your partner does, 90
  of new things to try, 91–2
locations for sex 57, 93, 177–8, 277–8
love
  find out who you're in love with, 174–5
  and good sex, 14, 142–4, 178–82, 263
  loving versus lusty sex, 40
lubricants, 92, 99, 102, 103, 105, 116, 139, 178, 191, 211,
  213–14, 226, 233, 235, 240

male contraception *see* condom, contraception
marriage
  affairs with married people, 256–7
  counselling, 275
  happiness and, 146–9
  median age of women's first, 13
  same sex, 250–1
  sex life and, 146–9, 264–5
  sexless, 146–9, 173, 212–18
massage, 203, 206
  deep tissue full-body, 217
  getting used to touch with, 62–3
  oil, 178
masturbation, 203, 209
  before sex, 19

effect on sex drive, 217
guilt about, 66
mutual, 118, 248
practising assessing arousal levels and, 114–15, 116
watching each other, 118, 190–2, 213
Matlock, Dr David, 141
menopause, 267
money and attraction, 139, 178
   see also social standing
monogamy
   attempted, 153
   is it too much to expect?, 150–2
   minuses, 152–3
   monotony of, 172–3
   plus points, 152
   points to negotiate, 152
   why?, 11–14
   see also infidelity
Morning After Pill (MAP), 32
   see also contraception
Morris, Desmond, 128, 132
multiple orgasms *see* orgasm
myths about sex, 68–72

new sexual techniques, 75–7
Nike approach to sex, 216
noisy sex, 256
norepinephrine, 286

O'Connell, Helen, 128
one night stands, 8–9
open relationships, 154–5
oral sex, 9, 50, 203, 211
   condoms and, 266
   gay, 248
   invention of, 78
   lesbian, 233
   married, 173
   practising, 76
   psychology of, 78

oral sex (*cont.*)
    shaving hair and, 266
    69er, 84, 113
    STIs and, 34, 35, 233
    swallowing sperm, 35, 85, 87, 233, 248
    time it takes a female to orgasm via, 44
    tips for females on giving great, 10, 83–7, 98
    tips for males on giving great, 11, 44, 78–83
orgasm
    anorgasmic, 211
    blended, 125
    breathing and, 124, 126, 240
    clitoral, 129, 130
    coital, 113
    coming together, 71–2, 112–19
    dizziness, headaches and, 268–9
    face, 122, 272–3
    female, evolutionary function of, 108–11
    female, genetic inheritance and, 111–12
    female failure to, 43–4
    female problems with, 211–12
    female via intercourse, 25
    female via oral sex, 82
    fingerprint, 124
    girl-on-girl, 233
    how long does it take a woman to?, 255, 279–80
    male failure to, 12, 24–26
    men rushing women to, 44
    multiple, 120–7, 121, 275
    non-ejaculatory (NEO), 120, 121, 122
    peaking techniques, 104, 125–6
    pre-orgasmic, 211
    should I leave if he can't give me an?, 163–4
    triggers, 126
    vaginal, 125
orgy *see* group sex
ovarian cysts, 212
oxytocin, 286–7

P-spot, 133–4

painful intercourse, 211–12
parents, effect on sex life, 61–7, 194
paying for sex, 19, 20–21, 257
PC (pubococcygeus) muscle, 25, 73, 117, 120, 123, 125, 140, 212
   see also Kegel exercises
peaking techniques, 104, 125–6
pelvic toners, 139–40
penis
   average, 41, 42
   and dildo, 234–5
   dreaming of, 145
   hardness of, 265
   head of, 210, 254–5
   large, 41–2, 77
   measuring, 42
   naming, 255–6
   small, 77, 254–5
   width, 41–2
   see also genitals
penis ring, 236, 283–4
performance, rating your, 38–9
perineum, 101, 117, 254
period, 128, 278–9
periurethral glands, 133
permission to explore your sexuality, giving yourself, 65–6
personality, sex and your, 4–5
pheromones, 28
phone sex, 188
PID (Pelvic Inflammatory Disease), 212
Pill, the
   Emergency (Morning After) Pill, 32, 33
   forgetting to take, 32–4
PMT (Pre-Menstrual Tension) 128
   see also period
pornography, 178, 188–9, 218
positions *see* intercourse
post-sex emotional fallout, 10
premature ejaculation, 19, 25, 209–10, 254–5, 258–9, 284
professional help, 61, 65
   see also therapists

prostate gland, 102, 134, 206, 209
prostitutes, 19, 20–2, 257
pubic hair, trimming, 265–6

questions, sex, 252–75
quickies, 91, 217–8

rape, 212
reading list, 289–91
rear-entry positions *see* intercourse
Relate, 206
relationships
    happiness and, 36
    makeover, 173–8
    open, 154–5
    problems with, 75
rimming, 35, 233, 248
role play, 177, 186–7
Rosen, Emanuel H., 197
rough sex, 40, 252–3

safe sex *see* contraception; STIs
scabies *see* genitals; STIs
scarves, 101, 178, 187
scent therapy, 140
Scentuelle, 140
Schnarch, David, 213–14
Secrets of Sexual Ecstasy (Broder and Goldman), 58
self-esteem, working on your, 68
self-image, female, 3, 10, 46–7
self-talk, be aware of, 67
semi-public sex, 177
Sensate Focus Programme, 206, 212
sensual massage *see* massage
serotonin, 130
settling down, why?, 11–14, 23, 273–4
    see also monogamy
sex
    distracted during, 262–3

good in bed checklist, 72–4
happiness and, 212–13
how good are you?, 38–9
how to appear better at, 51–7
inventory, 177
just to be polite, 274–5
long-term, 36–7, 174–82
quantum model, 213
rating partners, 49–51
spoil sessions, 177
sex aids or toys, 92, 178, 203, 281–6
    anal sex, 102, 104–6, 284
    dildos, 234–7, 281–3
    dress up clothes, 285
    lingerie for her, 285–6
    love balls, 283
    pelvic floor toners, 282
    penis rings, 236, 283–4
    S & M gear, 285
    STIs and, 34
    vibrating sleeves, 284–5
    whips, paddles and riding crops, 187, 285
    see also under individual toy
sex books, 58, 60, 61, 66
sex buddies, 7–8
Sex and the City, 8
sex contracts, 198–204, 215, 217
sex den, turn your bedroom into, 177–8
sex drive *see* libido, sexual arousal
Sex Inspectors, The, 76
sex saboteurs, 48, 59–68
    celebrities, 60–61
    exes, 59–60, 73
    family, 61–7
    friends, 61
Sex Smart: How Your Childhood Shaped Your Sexual Life and What to Do About It (Zoldbrod), 63, 64
sex therapist *see* therapists
sexual abuse, 212

sexual appetite, 36–7
sexual arousal, 114–15, 213–14
    see also arousal systems
sexual belief system, 58–68
sexual health clinics and check ups, 35–6, 212
Sexual Kung Fu, 123
sexuality, 223–5
shower, sex in, 278–9
side-by-side positions *see* intercourse
simultaneous orgasm *see* orgasm, coming together
singles life, 1–2, 11–14, 36–7
size of genitals and effect on sex life, 41–2, 77, 254–5
sleep
    masks, 178
    sex during, 93–4, 277–8
snog buddies, 7–8
social standing, 4, 139, 178
spanking, 177, 187, 248
spectatoring, stopping, 67
sperm 33, 85, 134, 232, 247
spiritual sex, 123
spontaneous sex, 49, 214
squeeze technique 210
STDs *see* STIs
STIs (sexually transmitted infections), 21, 34–6
    chlamydia, 35, 104
    gonorrhoea, 35, 104
    hepatitis, 35, 104, 233
    herpes, 35, 104, 233
    HIV/AIDS, 34, 35, 104, 233, 266
    HPV (genital warts), 35, 232
    pubic lice, 232
    same sex and, 232–3
    scabies, 232
    syphilis, 35
stockings, 178, 187
Stoppard, Miriam, 276
Story of O, 9
strangers, dreams of sex with, 146
strap-on dildos, 234–7

see also sex aids
stress, sex and, 10, 45, 202
supplements, 140
swinging, 154, 185–6

talking
    dirty, 91, 117, 177, 187–8
    using the right language, 196
    what you shouldn't say, 270–3
    women and, 158–60
testicles, 76, 85, 86, 101, 117, 190, 254, 265
    see also genitals
testosterone, 91
    boosters, 137, 138, 206
    and gay men and women, 238
texting, 90, 92, 149
    see also foreplay
therapists, 58, 63, 65, 116, 149, 192–3, 204–6, 212
therapy, DIY, 192–8, 204–12
threesomes, 185–6
tie-up games, 177, 178
tongue, 77, 78, 95
touching
    feeling uncomfortable with, 62–3
    techniques for, 102–4, 226
triphasic birth control pills, 140, 206
    see also contraception
trust, finding it hard to, 64–5
truthfulness about your past, 70–1

U-spot, 129–30
unresponsiveness *see* libido, sexual arousal
urethra, 129–30, 131, 134
useful contacts, 88–91

vacuum therapy, 137, 139, 208
vagina, 124
    complimenting her, 82–3
    front wall stimulation, 50, 117, 124, 129, 130–1, 131, 133,
        134, 163, 282

vagina (*cont.*)
    untoned, 207
    see also genitals
vaginal
    dilators, 140
    flowback, 109
    orgasms, 125
    see also genitals, STIs
vaginismus, 211–12
Viagra, 135–6, 137, 138
vibes, sending out sexual, 27–30, 244–5
vibrator, 122, 131, 163, 178, 191, 211, 218, 281–2
    A-spot, 133
    can they ruin sex?, 263–4
    invention of, 108, 109
    lesbians and, 233
    men and, 253–4
    'rabbit', 281
    strap-on, 231, 234–7
    wand, 45, 101, 115, 117, 253, 282
virginity, losing it, 49
    guide for him, 15–20, 63
    with a sex worker, 20–1
vulva, 129, 191

warts, genital, 34, 232
    see also genitals, STIs
websites, 35, 239, 281, 288–9
Whipple, Beverly, 88, 121
whips, 187, 285
Wilson, Dr Glenn, 93
withdrawal method, 33
    see also contraception
women on top positions *see* intercourse
workmates, sleeping with, 69–70
Would Like to Meet, 63
Wu Hu, 78

Zilbergeld, Bernie, 80, 270